DISEASES OF THE COLON AND RECTUM

with Self-assessment workbook

Ulcerative Colitis
Granulomatous Colitis
Diverticular Diseases of Colon
Cancer of Colon and Rectum

楊 謙 志

Him-che Yeung, L.Ac., O.M.D., Ph.D.

Copyright © 1993 by Institute of Chinese Medicine

All rights reserved. No part of this book shall be reproduced, stored in a retrieval system, or transmitted by any means, electronic, mechanical, photocopying, recording, without written permission from the publisher. Although every precaution has been taken in the preparation of this book, the author assume no responsibility for errors or omissions.

For information:
Institute of Chinese Medicine
602 San Gabriel Blvd., Rosemead, CA 91770
(818) 280-8811

International Standard Book Number: 0-9639715-0-6

Library of Congress Number: TXu 605 266

Printed in the United States of America

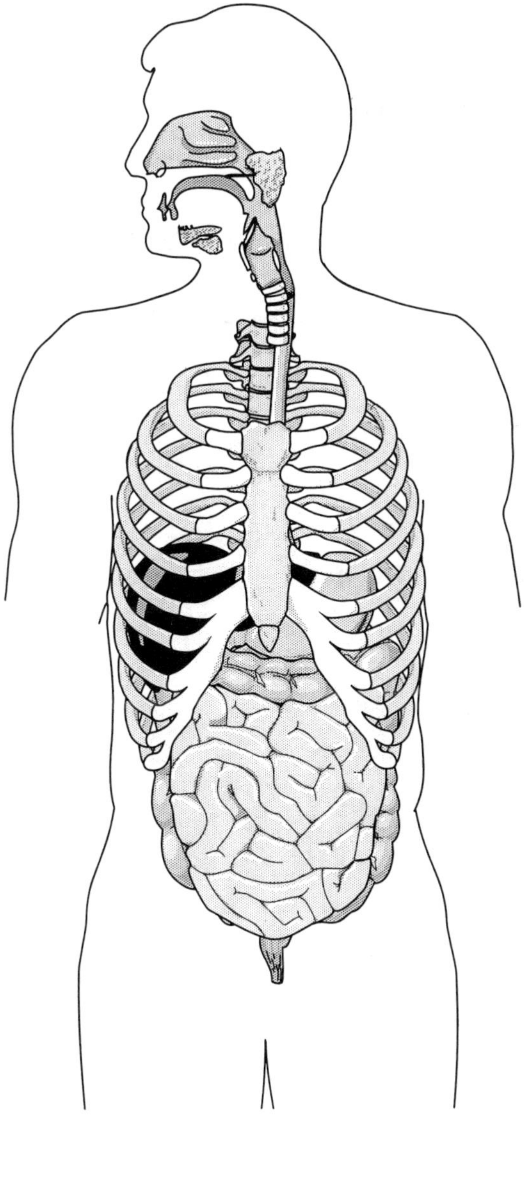

Acknowledgements

I am extremely grateful to the following personnels for their technical supports:

Maxwell Lee
Ke-xing Li
Steven Yu
Tuoc Kim Pham
Edward Tantraphol

Dedicated to all the physicians and health-care professionals who are interested in the ancient and modern methods of Chinese medical philosophy;

and to all the patients who are suffering from the ailments and are seeking for alternative methods of health care.

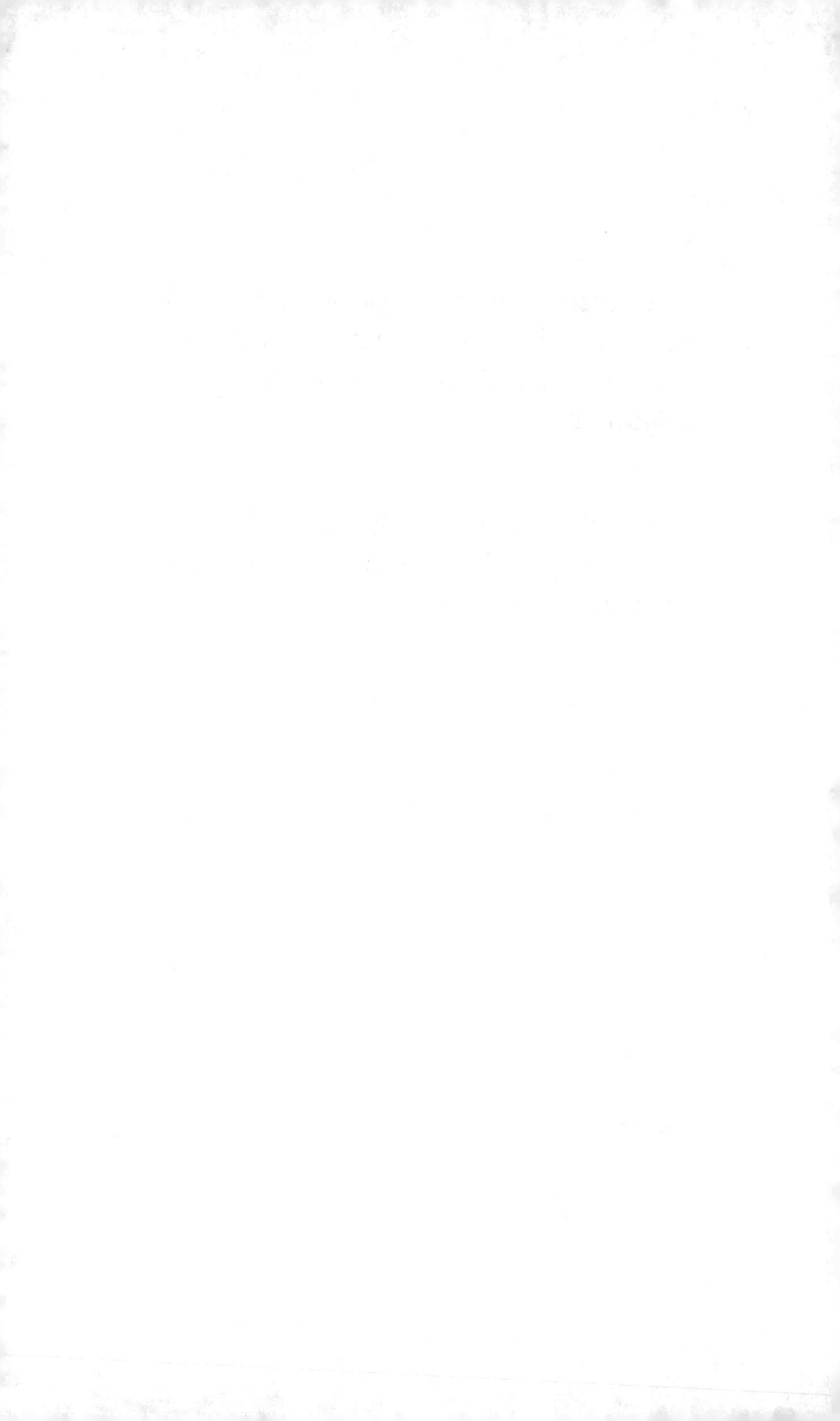

TABLE OF CONTENTS

Ulcerative Colitis 1
- Essentials of Diagnosis,1
- General Considerations,1
- Clinical Findings,2
- Differential Diagnosis,3
- Complications ,4
- Analysis and Pathogenesis (Chinese),5
- Chinese Differential Diagnosis,5
- Treatment (Chinese),6
- Treatment (Western),12
- Prevention,14
- Nutritional Care,14
- Chinese Diet Therapy,16

Granulomatous Colitis 21

Diverticular Diseases of Colon 22
- Essentials of Diagnosis,22
- General Considerations,22
- Clinical Findings,22
- Treatment,23

Cancer of Colon and Rectum 25
- Essentials of Diagnosis,25

General Considerations,25

Clinical Findings,26

Treatment,27

Chinese Methods of Differential Diagnosis and Treatment,28

Chemotherapy,30

Radiation Therapy,30

Fulguration,31

Integrated Chinese and Western Therapy,31

Nutritional Effects of Cancer Therapy,33

Nutritional Care of the Patients with Cancer,34

Chinese Herbs for Colon Cancer,36

Chinese Herbs for Colitis,52

Acupuncture Points Used,59

Glossary,74

Self-Assessment Workbook, 77

Index,88

THE LARGE INTESTINE

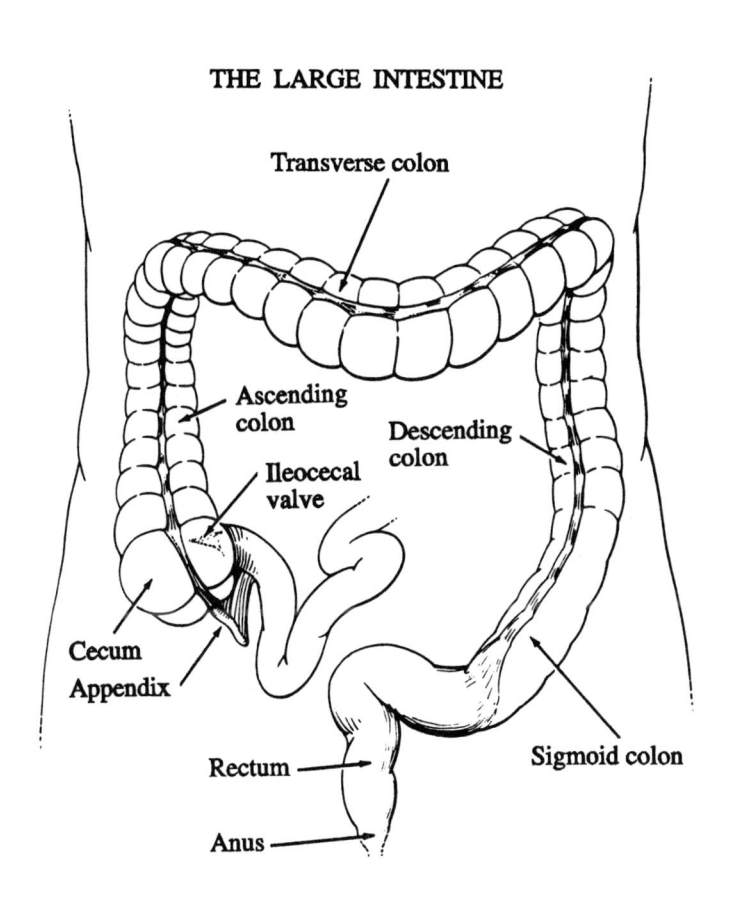

DISEASES OF THE COLON AND RECTUM

ULCERATIVE COLITIS

Essentials of Diagnosis:

- Bloody diarrhea with lower abdominal cramps.
- Mild abdominal tenderness, weight loss, fever.
- Anemia.
- Electrolyte imbalance.
- No stool pathogens.
- Specific X-ray and sigmoidoscopic abnormalities.

General Considerations:

Ulcerative colitis is also known as proliferative nonspecific ulcerative colitis. It is a persistent and recurring inflammatory disease of the colon of unknown causes. It is characterized by bloody diarrhea, tenesmus, abdominal pain, involving mainly of the left colon. It is primarily a disease of adolescents and adults between the age of 20 to 50.

The initial process may be acute or chronic inflmmation of the colon, with multiple irregular superficial ulceration. Repeated episodes lead to thickening of the walls with scar tissues. The proliferative changes in the epithelium may lead to polypoid structure. Pseudopolyps are indicative of severe ulceration.

This disease may be divided into 3 stages:

1. Mild case--most common. The initial process is slow and mild. Bloody diarrhea less than 5 times per day. The pathogenic sites are the colon and sigmoid colon.

2. Severe case -- Watery and bloody diarrhea over 5 times per day. Accompanied with fever, anemia and abdominal pain. Other complications such as toxic megacolon, acute proliferation of the colon, rectal or colon cancer, etc.

3. Severe (Fulminant) case -- Rare. Acute attack of the whole body, pain with oppression, hemorrhage, perforation, toxic megacolon, and sepsis developed over a short period of time. Cavities of the colon are acutely distended, with a diameter over 6 cm. May also have fever, increased palpitation, dehydration and prostration. The prognosis is very bad.

Clinical Findings:

A. **Symptoms and Signs**: Bloody diarrhea with blood and mucous in the stools, or blood and mucus may occur without feces. Constipation may occur instead of diarrhea. Nocturnal diarrhea may occur when daytime diarrhea is severe. Rectal tenesmus may be severe. Cramping lower abdominal pain often occurs. Anorexia, malaise, weakness and fatigue are also present. History of milk or dairy intolerance. There is a tendency toward remissions and exacerbation. Fever, weight loss and toxemia vary with the severity of the disease. Abdominal tenderness is generally mild. Abdominal distention may be present and is a poor prognostic sign.

B. **Laboratory Findings**: Hypochromic microcytic anemia is present due to blood loss. Stools contain blood, pus and mucus, but no pathogenic bacteria. Hypoproteinemia may occur. In severe situation, electrolyte disturbances is evident.

C. **X-ray Findings**: May vary from irritable and fuzzy margins to pseudopolyps, decreased size of colon, shortening and narrowing of the lumen, and loss of haustral markings.

D. **Colonoscopic Examination**: The mucosa is very swollen, increasing frangibility, and is friable when wiped with a cotton gauze. It varies from mucosal hyperemia, petechiae, and minimal granulation in mild cases to ulceration and polypoid changes in severe cases.

Differential Diagnosis:

1. Bacillary dysentery: abdominal pain and tenderness, blood and mucus in stool, tenesmus. Response to antibiotics. Stool culture is positive with Shigella dysentery.

2. Amoebic dysentery: Both right and side sides of the colon are affected. Cysts of the Entamoeba histolytica are found.

3. Schistosomiasis: Enlargement of the liver and spleen.

The ovum of the Schistosome parasite are found in the stool.

4. Colon cancer: Tumor may be palpated with rectal examination.

5. Enteric neurosis: Repeated lower abdominal pain with diarrhea or constipation. Stool with mucus, but no blood or pathogens. Normal barium enema and colonoscopic examination. Usually with heart palpitation, chest distress, dizziness, insomnia, worry, perspiration of the hands and feet.

6. Crohn's disease: Also known as granulomatous colitis. Distribution is segmental. Clinical manifestations are recurrent umbilical and right lower abdominal pain, diarrhea, no blood and mucus stool, no tenesmus, may have fever.

Complications:

1. Local Complications: include ischiorectal abscess, fistula, rectal prolapse, fibrous stricture of the rectum or colon, colonic perforation, carcinoma, and colonic hemorrhage.

2. Systemic Complications: include erythema nodosum, polyarthritis, ankylosing spondylitis, ocular lesions, conjunctivitis, liver diseases, anemia, thromophlebitis, etc.

Analysis and Pathogenesis (Chinese Medicine):

1. Accumulation of heat and dampness: Dampness is

accumulated either from exterior affection of pathogens, or imbalance of diet. Heat and fever is produced, and affecting the intestines.

2. Deficiency of the Spleen and Stomach: The spleen and stomach is upset by diet, causing the imbalance of digestion of food and grains, and the transportation of the molecules. Thus causing the reoccurrence of diarrhea and constipation.

3. Spleen is affected by Liver *Qi*: The spleen is affected by the emotion and neurosis which are controlled by the Liver *Qi*, thus affecting the function of the intestines.

4. Deficiency of Spleen and Kidney *Yang*: The digestion and transportation of the spleen is controlled by the Kidney *Yang* energy. If the Fire of Mingmen is diminished, then there is a malfunction in the reabsorption of water, thus causing diarrhea.

5. Stagnation of blood in the intestine meridian: Chronic heat and dampness are accumulated in the intestines, blocking the flow of energy in the intestine meridian. With the stagnation of flow of *Qi* and blood, blood and mucus are found in the stools.

Chinese Differential Diagnosis:

1. Diarrhea: Acute attack of diarrhea, with burning sensation in the anus is related to accumulation of Heat and Dampness. Chronic and recurrent diarrhea, affected by imbalance of diet, is related to weak spleen and stomach. If condition is affected by emotion and neurosis, is related to the affection of Liver *Qi*. If diarrhea is at night or early

morning, then the Spleen and Kidney are affected.

2. Stools: If the stool is loose and watery, thin white or thin mucus, it is related to cold and deficiency. If it is white and with sticky mucus, it is related to Heat and Deficiency. If the person has difficulty in bowel movement, or with blood and mucus, color is bright red, then is related to excessive heat syndromes.

3. Tenesmus: If tenesmus is relieved after bowel movement, it is related to Heat and Dampness. If tenesmus is not relieved after bowel movement, it is related to Spleen Deficiency. If tenesmus is accompanied with abdominal pain, and burning sensation in the anus, it is related to Heat and Fire. If abdominal pain is sharp, refused to be pressed, it is related to stagnation of Blood. If abdominal pain is cold, relieved by heat and pressure, it is related to Cold and Deficiency.

Treatment (Chinese):

1. Accumulation of Heat and Dampness: Stool with blood mucus, burning sensation in the anus, tenesmus with abdominal pain, refused to be pressed, may have fever, urination scanty and dark. Tongue red, with yellow and greasy coat. Pulse rapid and slippery.

Herbal Formulas: **Bai Tou Weng Tang**　白頭翁湯

白 頭 翁　Bai Tou Weng (Pulsatilla) *Radix Pulsatillae*
黃　　連　Huang Lian (Coptis) *Rhizoma Coptidis*
黃　　柏　Huang Bai (Phellodendron) *Cortex Phellodendri*
秦　　皮　Qin Pi (Fraxinus) *Cortex Fraxini*

白	芍	Bai Shao (White peony)	*Radix Paeoniae Alba*
木	香	Mu Xiang (Saussurea root)	*Radix Saussureae*

If heat is increased, add:

金 銀 花		Jin Yin Hua (Lonicera flower)	*Flos Lonicerae*
紅	藤	Hong Teng (Sargentodoxa stem)	*Caulis Sargentodoxae*
敗 醬 草		Bai Jiang Cao (Patrinia)	*Herba Patriniae*

If Dampness is increased, add:

蒼	朮	Cang Zhu (Atractylodes)	*Rhizoma Atractylodis*
厚	朴	Hou Po (Magnolia bark)	*Cortex Magnoliae Officinalis*
薏 苡 仁		Yi Yi Ren (Coix)	*Semen Coicis*
車 前 子		Che Qian Zi (Plantago seed)	*Semen Plantaginis*

With indigestion, abdominal pain, refused to be pressed, add:

檳	榔	Bing Lang (Areca seed)	*Semen Arecae*
枳	實	Zhi Shi (Immature bitter orange)	*Fructus Aurantii Immaturus*
山	楂	Shan Zha (Crataegus fruit)	*Fructus Crataegi*
神	曲	Shen Qu (Medicated leaven)	

2. Deficiency of Spleen and Stomach: Recurrent diarrhea, stool with white mucus or undigested food, abdominal pain is dull and prolonged, malaise, loss of appetite, distention after meal, color of face is sallow. Tongue pale with white coat. Pulse slow and weak.

Herbal Formula: **Shen Ling Bai Zhu San.** 參苓白朮散

人	參	Ren Shen (Ginseng) *Radix Ginseng*
蓮	子	Lian Zi (Lotus seed) *Semen Nelumbinis*
山	藥	Shan Yao (Dioscorea) *Rhizoma Dioscoreae*
白	朮	Bai Zhu (White atractylodes) *Radix Paeoniae Alba*
茯	苓	Fu Ling (Poria) *Poria*
白扁豆		Bai Bian Dou (Dolichos) *Semen Dolichi*
薏苡仁		Yi Yi Ren (Coix) *Semen Coicis*
砂	仁	Sha Ren (Cardamon) *Fructus Amomi*
桔	梗	Jie Geng (Platycodon) *Radix Platycodi*
甘	草	Gan Cao (Licorice) *Radix Glycyrrhizae*

With Dampness, add:

| 蒼 | 朮 | Cang Zhu (Atractylodes) *Rhizoma Atractylodis* |
| 厚 | 朴 | Hou Po (Magnolia bark) *Cortex Magnoliae Officinalis* |

With cold sensation, add:

| 附 | 子 | Fu Zi (Aconite) *Radix Aconiti Praeparata* |
| 乾 | 薑 | Gan Jiang (Dry ginger) *Rhizoma Zingiberis* |

With heat sensation, add:

| 黃 | 連 | Huang Lian (Coptis) *Rhizoma Coptidis* |
| 木 | 香 | Mu Xiang (Saussurea) *Radix Saussureae* |

With indigestion of food, add:

山	楂	Shan Sha (Crataegus) *Fructus Crataegi*
神	曲	Shen Qu (Medicated leaven) *Massa Fermentata Medicinalis*
雞內金		Ji Nei Jin (Gizzard skin) *Endothelium Corneum Gigeriae Galli*

With chronic diarrhea and deficiency of *Qi*, and prolapse, add:

| 黃 耆 | Huang Qi (Astragalus) *Radix Astragali* |
| 升 麻 | Sheng Ma (Cimicifuga) *Rhizoma Cimicifugae* |

3. Stagnation of Liver *Qi*: feeling of stuffiness and tightness in chest, belching, loss of appetite, abdominal pain and diarrhea after emotional upset or stimulation. Tongue pale red, thin coat. Pulse wiry.

Herbal Formulas: **Tong Xie Yao Fang**　痛瀉要方

白 术	Bai Zhu (White Atractylodes) *Rhizoma Atractylodis Macrophalae*
白芍藥	Bai Shao Yao (White peony) *Radix Paeoniae Alba*
陳 皮	Chen Pi (Citrus peel) *Pericarpium Citri Reticulatae*
防 風	Fang Feng (Ledebouriella) *Radix Ledebouriellae*

plus **Si Mo Yin**　四磨飲

人 參	Ren Shen (Ginseng) *Radix Ginseng*
檳 榔	Bing Lang (Areca seed) *Semen Arecae*
沉 香	Chen Xiang (Aquilaria wood) *Lignum Aquilariae Resinatum*
烏 藥	Wu Yao (Lindera root) *Radix Linderae*

4. Spleen and Kidney *Yang* Deficiency: Chronic diarrhea, abdominal pain and diarrhea in early morning, pain relieved after bowel movement, low back pain, abdomen and the extremities with cold sensation, fatigue. Tongue pale with thin white coat. Pulse deep and thready.

Herbal Formulas: **Fu Zi Li Zhong Wan**　附子理中丸

| 附 子 | Fu Zi (Aconite) *Radix Aconiti Praeparata* |

人 參	Ren Shen (Ginseng) *Radix Ginseng*
白 朮	Bai Zhu (White Atractylodes) *Rhizoma Atractylodis Macrocephalae*
乾 薑	Gan Jiang (Dry Ginger) *Rhizoma Zingiberis*
甘 草	Gan Cao (Baked Licorice) *Radix Glycyrrhizae*

plus **Si Shen Wan** 四神丸

補骨脂	Bu Gu Zhi (Psoralea) *Fructus Psoraleae*
吳茱萸	Wu Zhu Yu (Evodia) *Fructus Evodiae*
肉豆蔻	Rou Dou Kou (Nutmeg) *Semen Myristicae*
五味子	Wu Wei Zi (Schisandra) *Fructus Schisandrae*
生 薑	Sheng Jiang (Fresh Ginger) *Rhizoma Zingiberis Recens*
大 棗	Da Zao (Jujube) *Fructus Ziziphus Jujubae*

If diarrhea is excessive, add:

| 赤石脂 | Chi Shi Zhi (Red hallocysite) *Halloysitum rubrum* |
| 訶 子 | He Zi (Terminalia fruit) *Fructus Terminaliae* |

5. Stagnation of Blood in the Intestine Meridian: Chronic diarrhea, stool with bloody mucus, abdomen with sharp pain, very painful on pressure, face with dim and black complexion. Tongue dark red with red spots, with white coat. Pulse thready or hesistant.

Herbal Formula: **Shao Fu Zhu Yu Tang** 少腹逐瘀湯

| 當 歸 | Dang Gui (Chinese Angelica) *Radix Angelicae Sinensis* |
| 川 芎 | Chuan Xiong (Ligusticum) *Rhizoma Ligustici Chuanxiong* |

赤芍藥　Chi Shao Yao (Red peony) *Radix Paeoniae Rubra*

小茴香　Xiao Hui Xiang (Fennel) *Fructus Foeniculi*

延胡索　Yan Hu Suo (Corydalis) *Rhizoma Corydalis*

五靈脂　Wu Ling Zhi (Trogopterus) *Faeces Trogopterorum*

沒　藥　Mo Yao (Myrrh) *Resina Myrrhae*

肉　桂　Rou Gui (Cinnamon Bark) *Cortex Cinnamomi*

乾　薑　Gan Jiang (Dry Ginger) *Rhizoma Zingiberis*

蒲　黃　Pu Huang (Bulrush pollen) *Pollen Typhae*

Enema Therapy (Chinese)

1. **Xi Lei San**　錫類散

1 gm. of **Sheng Ji San**　生肌散

爐甘石　Lu Gan Shi (Calamine) *Calamina*

鍾乳石　Zhong Ru Shi (Stalactite) *Stalactitum*

琥　珀　Hu Po (Amber) *Succinum*

滑　石　Hua Shi (Talc) *Talcum*

硃　砂　Zhu Sha (Cinnabar) *Cinnabaris*

冰　片　Bing Pian (Borneol) *Borneolum*

and 1 gm. of **Yun Nan Bai Yao** 雲南白藥 (Chinese patent formula) to 100 c.c. of warm water.

2. Alum Compound (**Ming Fan He Ji**)　明礬合劑

明　礬　Ming Fan (Alum) *Alumen*

蒼　朮　Cang Zhu (Atractylodes) *Rhizoma Atractylodis*

苦　參　Ku Shen (Sophora) *Radix Sophorae Flavescentis*

槐　花　Huai Hua (Sophora) *Flos Sophorae*

Add 15 gm of above ingredients to 10 gm. of

大　黃　Da Huang (Rhubarb) *Radix et Rz. Rhei*

Add water to boil down to 250 c.c. of water. Use 50 - 80 c.c. each time for enema.

Acupuncture Treatments:

Zhongwan (Ren 12) 中脘, Zusanli (St. 36) 足三里, Tianshu (St. 25) 天樞, Dachangshu (U.B. 25) 大腸俞. With weak Spleen and Stomach, add Pishu (U.B. 20) 脾俞 and Weishu (U.B. 21) 胃俞, Zhangmen (Liv. 13) 章門, and Qihai (Ren 6) 氣海. With Spleen and Kidney *Yang* Deficiency, add Shenque (Ren 8) 神闕, Guanyuan (Ren 4) 關元, Shenshu (U.B. 23) 腎俞, and Mingmen (Du 4) 命門. Each time select 3 to 4 points, alternate using the points. May use moxibustion after acupuncture needle therapy. Shenque (Ren 8) 神闕 point may use indirect moxibustion with ginger or aconite daily. Other points may use moxibustion with moxa sticks or wools, or indirectly with ginger.

Treatment (Western):

A. Severe (fulminant) condition:

　1. Hospitalization

　2. General measures:

　　a. Increase blood volume with fluids, plasma or blood. With excessive bleeding, use hemostatic.

- b. Correct electrolyte abnormalities, especially potassium supplement.
- c. Discontinue all oral intake. Start nasogastric suction if the colon has become dilated.
3. Antimicrobial therapy - With peripheral infection or toxemia, use antibiotics such as ampicillin, cephalothin, chloramphenicol, and gentamicin.
4. Adrenocorticosteroid - Give intravenous dosage of hydrocortisone (300 mg. dosage daily, prednisolone-21-phosphate (60 mg daily) in divided doses at 6-hr intervals.
5. Surgery - colonic resection or colectomy.

B. Moderate condition: patients do not have severe Hypoproteinemia, fever or leukocytosis.
1. Antimicrobial therapy - Sulfasalazine, 2-4 gm daily in 3 divided doses.
2. Adrenocorticosteroid - Prednisone 20-40 mg orally daily. Reduce 5 mg per day per week slowly to 10-15 mg daily.
3. Diet: no milk or dairy products. All food must be cooked.

C. Mild condition: patients with minimal inflammation, and no systemic signs of the disease.
1. Antimicrobial therapy - Sulfasalazine 2-4 gm daily in divided doses.
2. Adrenocorticosteroid - Hydrocortisone enemas, 100 mg each night until lesion heals, or condition is stabilized.
3. Diet - no milk and dairy products.

Prevention:

1. When diarrhea with bloody stools is frequent, try bed rest. Average patients can do *Qi Gong* and *Tai Qi* breathing exercises to strengthen the body.

2. Keep the living environment clean and peaceful, so the patient can keep calm and peaceful. Avoid emotional stress and tension.

3. Keep the body warm. Avoid catching a cold. Spleen and Kidney *Yang* deficiency patients with abdominal pain may use hot pad to keep the abdomen warm. The temperature of the fluids used for enema may be kept at 38 to 40°C.

4. Keep the underwear and bed sheets clean and dry. Pay attention to the hygiene of the skin around the hip. Avoid prolapse.

Nutritional Care:

1. Keep a high protein, high calorie diet, low in fiber and rich in vitamins and nutrients. Moderately sick patients need to be on liquid or semi-liquid diet. Avoid cold, spicy, greasy, spoiled or other stimulatory foods. Porridge, soup cooked with bones or eggs, and soft noodles made good semi-liquid diet. Slow cookers made excellent porridge of different kinds and soups with bones.

2. If iron is indicated to correct anemia, it should be given intramuscularly to avoid irritation of the mucus and the poor absorption of iron.

3. If megaloblastic anemia is present, it should be

determined whether the anemia is due to folate or vitamin B_{12} deficiency. Sulfasalazine is known to decrease absorption of folate.

4. Total parenteral nutrition (TPN) may be necessary if the patient cannot absorb nutrients or if food exacerbates the diarrhea. In enteral feeding, a 3-day trial with oral feeding that is carefully monitored. If the patient cannot ingest 1000 to 1500 kcal. per day, then tube feeding should be started.

5. Milk allergy is frequently found in these patients, so it is wise to limit milk intake. It is best to first establish whether there is a lactose intolerance by appropriate testing, and if so, lactase can be added to milk or milk products. A diet free of lactose may be helpful to the intolerant patients. Ice cream is sometimes used to help calories to the diet.

6. The intake of high doses of antibiotics may upset the normal bacterial flora in the intestines. Plenty of yogurt, whey powder and acidophilus culture may be given to restore the proper bacterial balance in the intestines. Whey is the residue from milk after removal of casein and fat, also known as lacto-serum.

7. Hi-fiber substances should be eliminated from the patient suffering from any form of diarrhea. Many high-fiber substances are high-roughage substances are bland. Daikon, garlic, persimmon and black fungus is good for diarrhea condition. If diarrhea is severe, frequent drinking of dark green tea is helpful. Tea and persimmon contain tannin which is an astringent.

8. Besides a low-fiber diet, it is good to eat a variety of

food at any meal. Often patients can tolerate small feedings whereas a very large meal will induce more peristaltic activity. Very cold foods may induce peristalsis as opposed to room-temperature or slightly warm foods.

9. Lotus root or hot drinks made from the dry powder can help to relieve the bloody stools. Dissolve two tablespoons of lotus powder with 1 tabs of cold water, mix with a spoon until all the powder turned into a paste form. Add boiling water to the cup slowly, and stirring constantly as you add the hot water. Lotus root contains tannin and asparagine. It can be used to lower the temperature in the blood, stop bleeding and eliminate stagnation.

10. Restriction of whole grains and whole products, which if not properly digested, can cause fermentation in the bowels, with consequent gas and bowel irritation. If the action of fermentation is strong in the intestines, eat food with protein and less fat, such as dairy products, eggs, soy milk. Avoid sugar which can produce gas and fermentation. If the petrification is strong in the intestines, eat more starch products such as potatoes, taro, rice and flours. Reduce intake of meat, egg, fish or bean with high proteins.

11. Supplement intake of high vitamin-C drinks, such as orange juice, fresh tomato juice, vegetable juice, or fortified vitamin-C drinks.

12. Avoid alcohol, coffee, chocolate, cold tea, soft drinks, spices, pepper, mustard, curry, hard or high cellulose fruits and vegetables. Bananas are very soothing and healing in ulcerative colitis. Millet cereal is best. Sprouted seeds and grains are usually well tolerated. All foods must be eaten slowly, chewed and salivated well. Eat 3-5 small meals per day is preferred.

Chinese Diet Therapy:

1. Dioscorea cake:

Ingredients:

250 gm. Fresh dioscorea (Shan Yao) 山藥 *Rhizoma Dioscoreae*
150 gm. Adsuki bean (Chi Xiao Dou) 赤小豆 *Semen Phaseoli*
30 gm. Euryale seed (Qian Shi) 芡實 *Semen Euryales*
20 gm. Dolichos seed (Bai Bian Dou) 白扁豆 *Semen Dolichi*
20 gm. Poria (Fu Ling) 茯苓 *Poria*
4 pc. Black plums (Wu Mei) 烏梅 *Fructus Mume*
Fruit cocktail

Method of Preparation:

Grind the adsuki bean into paste, and mix with small amount of sugar. Grind the poria, dolichos seed, and euryale into fine powder. Steam with small amount of water. Peel the skin of the freshly steamed dioscorea, and mix with the poria powder into a paste. Brush one layer of dioscorea powder, and one layer of adsuki bean paste. Repeat several times with the layering. On the top layer, add some fruit cocktail. Steam for app. 15 min. Make a syrup with the black plums and sugar. Pour over the cake.

2. Baked spicy chicken:

Ingredients:

750 gm. Sliced chicken
6 gm. Dry ginger
3 gm. Evodia (Wu Zhu Yu) 吳茱萸 *Fructus Evodiae*

3 gm.   Nutmeg (Rou Dou Kou)   肉豆蔻 *Semen Myristicae*
2 gm.   Cinnamon bark (Rou Gui)   肉桂 *Cortex Cinnamomi*
1 gm.   Cloves (Ding Xiang)   丁香 *Flos Caryophylli*
Soy sauce
Cooking wine
Sugar

Method of Preparation:

Grind the dry ginger, evodia, nutmeg, cloves and cinnamon bark into powder. Add soy sauce, cooking wine, sugar, and mix with the herb powder. Rub the chicken with the herb powder, and marinate for 3 hours. Put the chicken into the oven and bake for 15 min. Turn over the chicken and bake for another 15 minutes.

3. Sweetened persimmon and longan fruit cake:

Ingredients:

500 gm. Persimmon cake
20 pc. Longan (Gui Yuan) 桂圓 *Arillus Longan*
15 gm. Codonopsis (Dang Shen) 黨參 *Radix Codonopsis Pilosulae*
15 gm. Astragalus (Huang Qi) 黃耆 *Radix Astragali*
20 gm. Dioscorea (Shan Yao) 山藥 *Rhizoma Dioscoreae*
20 gm. Lotus seed (Lian Zi) 蓮子 *Semen Nelumbinis*
Honey
Brown Sugar

Method of Preparation:

Slice each persimmon cake into 4 pieces. Remove the peel and seed of the longan. Crush the codonopsis and astragalus. Peel the dioscorea, and cut into slices. Remove the plummule of the lotus seed. Add the above ingredients into a clay pot. Add honey, brown sugar and water. Steam for 2-3 hours. It can get very thick like a syrup. Ready to eat when it is cool. Eat 1-2 tablespoon each time, 2-3 times per day.

4. Porridge with lychee, dioscorea and lotus seed:

Ingredients:

50 gm. Dry lychee fruit 荔枝
10 gm. Dioscorea (Shan Yao) 山藥 *Rhizoma Dioscoreae*
10 gm. Lotus seed (Lian Zi) 蓮子 *Semen Nelumbinis*
50 gm. Rice (short-grain)

Method of Preparation:

Grind the dry lychee fruit, dioscorea, and lotus seed. Mix with rice in the rice cooker. Add 4 cups of water. Cook for app. 45 min. into porridge. Eat everyday.

5. Leek, ginger and milk juice:

Ingredients:

250 gm. Leek
25 gm. Fresh ginger
250 c.c. Milk

Method of Preparation:

Wash the leek and fresh ginger. Cut or grind into small pieces. Wrap with a piece of clean cheesecloth, and squeeze out the juice. Mix the juice with the milk and boil the mixture. Drink while it is hot. Drink 2 cups per day for several days.

6. Pomegranate syrup:

Ingredients:

1000 gm. Fresh pomegranate peel
300 gm. Honey

Method of Preparation:

Clean the pomegranate, and peel the skin. Cut the peel into small pieces. Add water and boil. Every 30 min. get the extract. Add more water to the peel, and boil for another 30 min. Mix the previous extract together. Simmer until the herb becomes concentrated. Add honey and boil. Pour the syrup into jars when it is cold. Take 1 tbsp. each times, and twice daily with boiling water.

GRANULOMATOUS COLITIS

(Crohn's Disease of the Colon)

Crohn's granulomatosis (Transmural colitis) is difficult to distinguish from the mucosal microabscess of colitis (ulcerative colitis). The distinguished feature is the transmural involvement in Crohn's colitis. It involves all layers of the bowel wall, including the serosa. The external surface displays serositis and appears erythematous. The intestinal wall is thickened due to lymphatic dilation and edema. The mucosa is red and swollen, with the presence of ulcerative lesions. Ulcers penetrate into the submucosa or deeper. Fissures penetrate the bowel wall, leading to the formation of fistulas and abscesses. Granulomas are seen in most of the pathology specimens. In the later stages, edematous bowel wall may be replaced by rigid fibrous tissues and gets thicker. This may lead to chronic intestinal obstruction and loss of anal sphincter function.

The most common clinical manifestations are abdominal cramps, diarrhea, and weight loss. Patients have less rectal bleeding and more tenesmus. Abdominal distention and tenderness usually in the right lower quadrant. The stool may be positive for occult blood.

The treatment of granulomatous colitis is essentially the same as for idiopathic ulcerative colitis. Patients should be started on Sulfasalazine or Prednisone. There is no advantage in using both drugs simultaneously. Dehydration should be corrected with intravenous fluids.

DIVERTICULAR DISEASE OF THE COLON

Essentials of Diagnosis:

- Intermittent, left lower abdominal pain with cramps.
- Constipation, or alternating constipation and diarrhea.
- Tenderness in the left lower quadrant.

General Considerations:

Diverticulitis of the colon occur primarily in the pressure areas of the colon. They tend to dissect along the course of the nutrient vessels. They are most common in the sigmoid colon and occur with increasing frequency after age 40. Inflammation vary from mild infiltration in the wall of the sac to the surrounding area, with perforation or abscess.

Urinary frequency and dysuria may occur if the inflammation involves the bladder. Red and white blood cells may be seen in the urine.

Clinical Findings:

A. **Symptoms and Signs**: Left lower quadrant abdominal pain with intermittent cramps, relieved by a bowel movement. Constipation, or alternating constipation and diarrhea. In some cases, occult blood is found in the stool. Massive hemorrhage may occur and causes colonic hemorrhage.

B. **X-ray Findings**: X-ray examination reveals diverticula, thickened interhaustral folds and narrowed colonic lumen.

Treatment:

1. Antibiotics (ampicillin, cephalothin, penicillin and streptomycin) are used in acute diverticulitis.

2. Presence of perforation, fistula or abscess will require surgical resection of the involved portion of the colon.

3. A diet high in residue.

4. Psyllium seed as bulk additives.

5. Add 1/4 cup of unprocessed bran in fruit juice or applesauce. Olive oil, mineral oil, and vegetable gum laxatives may be used. Bran intake should be started slowly. A rapid increase in bran intake can cause abdominal distention and pain. Patients should start with 1 tsp./day and increase to 8 or 10 tsp./day.

6. If constipation is the predominant symptom, high-fiber diet and high bran are indicated. The use of laxatives should be a last resort.

7. If diarrhea is the predominant symptom, the high-fiber diet is tried first. If it fails, a more bland, soft diet is used.

8. If pain is the predominant symptom, anticholinergic is given.

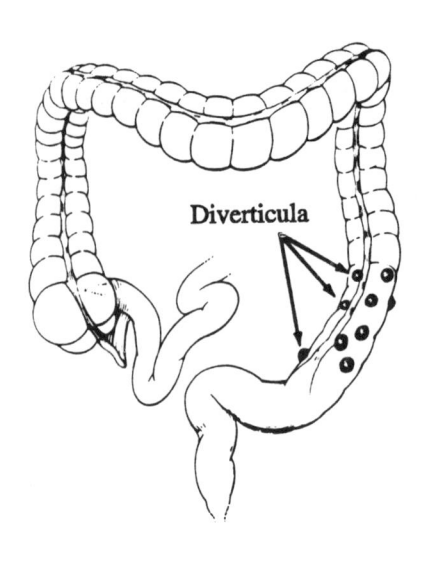

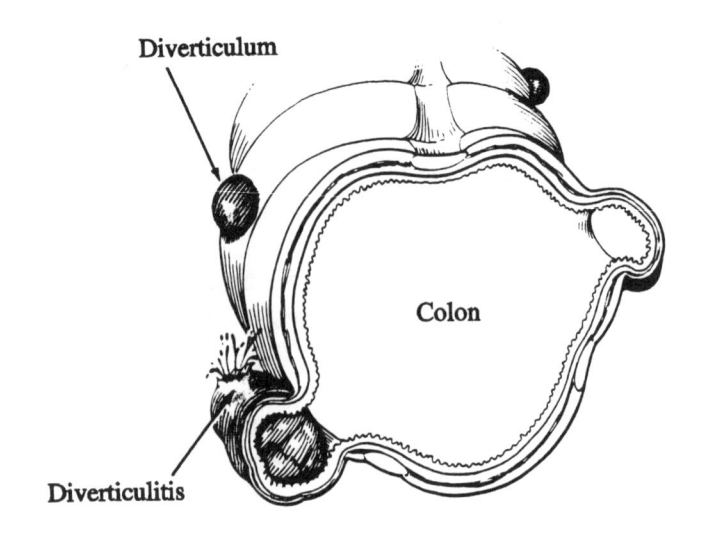

Diverticula are small pouches of the large intestine. If the diverticula become inflammed or ruptured, the condition is called diverticulitis.

CARCINOMA OF THE COLON AND RECTUM

Essentials of Diagnosis:

- Altered constipation or diarrhea
- Palpable mass involving colon or rectum
- Blood in the stools
- Weight loss
- Unexplained weight loss
- Sigmoidoscopic or X-ray showing neoplasm

General Considerations:

Carcinoma of the colon and rectum causes more death than other kinds of cancer. Males are affected more than female in a ratio of 3:2. Patients are usually over 50 years old. 50% of the cancer are found in the rectum, 20% in the sigmoid, 15% in the cecum and ascending colon, the rest in the transverse and descending colon. Carcinoma of the colon is related to the population with high fat, high beef and low fiber diet. The increase of bile acid and cholesterol in the intestine changes the normal flora, and increase of anaerobic bacillus. The evacuation time is prolonged in the intestine because of the low fiber diet, the cancer causing agents have more contact with the mucosa and cause cancer. Also in the regions with low selenium in the soil, cancer of the colon is also increased. Study of the genetics of the patients with cancer of colon have found that they have a history of adenomatous polyp of colon, osteoma and cancer of soft tissue.

Clinical Findings:

There is a change in the regular bowel movements. Bleeding and blood in the stools. Perforation or colonic obstruction may cause an acute attack on the abdomen. Sigmoidoscopy and X-ray show evidence of the cancer.

A. Cancer of the right colon: Usually belongs to medullary carcinoma. Because the bowel lumen is larger in the right half of the colon, and the feces are more liquid, there is less frequency of bowel obstruction. Vague abdominal discomfort may progress to cramping pain. There is unexplained anemia, weakness and weight loss. Stools are positive for occult blood. Palpable mass is found in the right lower quadrant. Bowel movement is more diarrhea.

B. Cancer of the left colon: Usually belongs to fibrocarcinoma. Because the lumen of the left side is narrower than the right side, stools are already formed. Thus bowel movement is more of constipation than diarrhea, occasionally with small amount of blood. There is acute colonic obstruction with abdominal pain and distention. Abdominal metallic sound or gurgling sound may be present. Palpable mass is present in the left lower quadrant. Anemia, weakness and weight loss are found. If obstruction is prolonged, a series of toxic symptoms or coma may happen.

C. Cancer of the rectum: The chief symptoms are bloody stools with increase of bowel movements, pain in the anus, tenesmus, and difficulty in passing feces. The color of the blood may be bright red or purplish red, with increase of mucous. When the peripheral tissues or the sacral plexus are invaded by the tumors, it will cause local sharp pain radiating to the abdomen and sacral area. When the tumor affects the bladder and prostate, bloody stools, frequency of urination and difficulty in urination may be resulted. If the vagina is affected, the female patient will have leukorrhea. Vaginal recto-fistula may be formed at the late stage.

D. Cancer of the anus: With chronic fistula, the symptoms of pain around the anus, with increase pain in defecation, and bright red bloody stool. If the tumor invades the anal sphincter, symptoms of fecal incontinence will occur. Large and hard inguinal lymph nodes can be palpated with metastasis.

The routes of metastasis are through the spread of blood flow, lymph nodes, and direct infiltration through the serous membrane into the neighboring organs such as the ureter, uterus and urinary bladder.

In the later stage of colon cancer, there is difficulty in urination, palpable mass in the abdomen, hepatomegaly, hepatitis, ascites, intestinal obstruction, enlarged lymph nodes above the left clavicle.

Treatment (Western):

The only cure for cancer of the large bowel is surgical resection of the lesion. It can relieve obstruction, bleeding, and symptoms of local invasion. There is 50% chance of survival over 5 years.

Treatment and Differential Diagnosis (Chinese):

1. Accumulation of Heat and Dampness: Intermittent abdominal pain, tenesmus, thirsty, fullness in the chest, nausea, poor appetite, diarrhea with blood and mucus. Tongue with thick yellow coat. Pulse is rapid and slippery.

Formula: **Modified Huai Jiao Wan**　加減槐角丸

槐 花	Huai Hua (Sophora flower) *Flos Sophorae*
地 瑜	Di Yu (Sanguisorba root) *Radix Sanguisorbae*
白 頭 翁	Bai Tou Weng (Pulsatilla) *Radix Pulsatillae*
敗 醬 草	Bai Jiang Cao (Patrinia) *Herba Patriniae*
馬 齒 莧	Ma Chi Xian (Portulaca) *Herba Portulacae*
黃 芩	Huang Qin (Scutellaria) *Radix Scutellariae*
黃 柏	Huang Bai (Phellodendron) *Cortex Phellodendri*
薏 苡 仁	Yi Yi Ren (Coix) *Semen Coicis*
枳 殼	Zhi Ke (Bitter orange) *Fructus Aurantii*
甘 草	Gan Cao (Licorice root) *Radix Glycyrrhizae*

2. Stagnation of Blood and *Qi* (Vital Energy): Abdominal distention with sharp pain, mass is firm and non-movable, tenesmus, diarrhea with dark purplish red blood. Tongue color dark purplish or with blood spots, with yellow coat. Pulse is hesitant.

Formula: **Modified Ge Xia Zhu Yu Tang**　膈下逐瘀湯

| 當 歸 | Dang Gui (Chinese angelica) *Radix Angelicae* |
| 赤 芍 藥 | Chi Shao Yao (Red peony) *Radix Paeoniae Rubra* |

紅	花	Hong Hua (Safflower)	*Flos Carthami*
桃	仁	Tao Ren (Persica seed)	*Semen Persicae*
枳	殼	Zhi Ke (Bitter orange)	*Fructus Aurantii*
烏	藥	Wu Yao (Lindera root)	*Radix Linderae*
牡丹皮		Mu Dan Pi (Moutan bark)	*Cortex Moutan Radicis*
金銀花		Jin Yin Hua (Lonicera flower)	*Flos Lonicerae*
延胡索		Yan Hu Suo (Corydalis)	*Rhizoma Corydalis*
忍冬藤		Ren Dong Teng (Lonicera stem)	*Caulis Lonicerae*
甘	草	Gan Cao (Licorice root)	*Radix Glycyrrhizae*

3. In the later stage of the disease, the patient get to be very weak. With Deficiency of *Yang* of Spleen and Kidney, use

Shen Ling Bai Zhu San　參苓白朮散

plus **Si Shen Wan**　四神丸

With Deficiency of *Yang* of Liver and Kidney, use

Zhi Bai Di Huang Wan　知柏地黃丸

With Deficiency of both *Qi* (vital energy) and Blood, use

Ba Zhen Tang　八珍湯

4. In general, if cancer cells are proliferative, add:

白花蛇舌草 Bai Hua She She Cao (Oldenlandia)
　　　　　Herba Oldenlandiae

半　枝　蓮　Ban Zhi Lian (Barbat skullcap)
　　　　　Herba Scutellariae Barbatae

敗醬草　Bai Jiang Cao (Patrinia herb) *Herba Patriniae*

苦　參　Ku Shen (Sophora root) *Radix Sophorae Flavescentis*

With tenesmus, add:

黃　連　Huang Lian (Coptis) *Rhizoma Coptidis*

木　香　Mu Xiang (Saussurea root) *Radix Saussureae*

With bloody stools, add:

地　瑜　Di Yu (Sanguisorba root) *Radix Sanguisorbae*

側柏葉　Ce Bai Ye (Biota tops) *Cacumen Biotae*

With abdominal pain, add:

烏　藥　Wu Yao (Lindera root) *Radix Linderae*

With abdominal distention, add:

枳　殼　Zhi Ke (Bitter orange) *Fructus Aurantii*

厚　朴　Hou Po (Magnolia bark) *Cortex Magnoliae Officinalis*

Chemotherapy:

Cytotoxic drugs such as 5-Fluouracil (5-Fu) is the first choice for colorectal cancer in the preoperative period. The standard treatment consist of intravenous administration for 5 consecutive days, once daily. Repeat after one month.

Radiation Therapy:

Today's modern instruments have energy sources of 1 million volts or more. This energy can be focused on deep-seated tumors, while sparing the skin and subcutaneous tissues and thus avoiding the severe desquamation characteristic of low-voltage radiation therapy. Preoperative irradiation is beneficial for patients with a small tumor, because the size of the tumor can be reduced, making it easier for surgical removal. Postoperative irradiation is recommended for stage B and stage C of rectal cancers. Unfortunately, it cannot prevent the spread of cancer during pelvic dissection nor does it protect the normal segment of bowel from the long-term adverse effects of irradiation, which can include proctitis, stricture, and fistula formation.

Fulguration (Elector-cauterization):

Elector-cauterization is used more for polypoid adenocarcinoma. If the patient is very old, very weak, or because of other conditions, or refused to have surgery, this is a method of choice.

Integrated Chinese and Western Therapy:

Colorectal cancer should be surgical removed in the initial stage of tumor. Combining Chinese herbs with western chemotherapy and radiation therapy can increase the effect of therapy. Chemotherapy and radiation therapy can lower the personal defense mechanism during the period. The wbc and platelets are usually decreased. The adverse effects of 5-Fu is diarrhea, vomiting, abdominal pain and suppression of the bone marrow. The Chinese herbs can enhance the immune system, stimulate the reticulo-endothelial system, regulate the metabolism of the connective tissue, and eliminate fibrosis caused by radiation.

1. For patients with symptoms of dry mouth and throat, constipation, irritable, urination dark, poor appetite, use:

生地黃	Sheng Di Huang (Raw Rehmannia) *Radix Rehmanniae*
沙參	Sha Shen (Glehnia root) *Radix Glehniae*
麥門冬	Mai Men Dong (Ophiopogon root) *Radix Ophiopogonis*
天花粉	Tian Hua Fen (Trichosanthes) *Radix Trichosanthis*
白茅根	Bai Mao Gen (Imperata rhizome) *Rhizoma Imperata*

2. For patients with symptoms of nausea, vomiting, constipation, lack of appetite, use:

黨參	Dang Shen (Codonopsis) *Radix Codonopsis Pilosulae*
白朮	Bai Zhu (White Atractylodes) *Rz Atractylodis Macrocephalae*
砂仁	Sha Ren (Cardamon) *Fructus Amomi*
竹茹	Zhu Ru (Bamboo shavings) *Caulus Bambusae in Taenis*
半夏	Ban Xia (Pinellia) *Rhizoma Pinelliae*
生薑	Sheng Jiang (Fresh ginger) *Rhizoma Zingiberis Recens*

3. For patients with symptoms of dizziness, malaise, stomach vertigo, severe palpitation, nose bleeding, skin with purpura, decreased WBC and platelets, use:

黃耆	Huang Qi (Astragalus root) *Radix Astragali*
當歸	Dang Gui (Chinese Angelica) *Radix Angelicae Sinensis*
雞血藤	Ji Xue Teng (Millettia) *Caulis Milletti*

大	棗	Da Zao (Chinese date) *Fructus Ziziphus Jujubae*
黃	精	Huang Jing (Solomonseal) *Rhizoma Polygonati*
枸杞子		Gou Qi Zi (Wolfberry fruit) *Fructus Lycii*
何首烏		He Shou Wu (Fleeceflower) *Radix Polygoni Multiflori*
紫河車		Zi He Che (Human placenta) *Placenta Hominis*

4. Acupuncture treatment on the following points:

上巨虛		Shangjuxu (St. 37)
大腸俞		Dachangshu (U.B. 25)
腎	俞	Shenshu (U.B. 23)
脾	俞	Pishu (U.B. 20)
關	元	Guanyuan (Ren 4)
合	谷	Hegu (L.I. 4)

Aquapuncture with Vit. B_{12} on the acupuncture points can increase the wbc and rbc and increase the immune system.

Nutritional Effects of Cancer Therapy:

Chemotherapy: Food intake is inhibited by the mucositis, cheilosis, glossitis, stomatitis and esophagitis caused by many drugs. Nausea and vomiting occur with almost all antineoplastic drugs. Abnormal taste sensation leads to anorexia and oligophagy (eating few foods). Diarrhea may be induced or there may be constipation or inhibition of bowel motility.

Radiation Therapy: Radiation of the upper part of the body may produce sore throat, mucositis, xerostomia (mouth dryness), and altered taste and smell. Radiation to the abdomen may produce acute gastritis or enteritis with nausea, vomiting, diarrhea and anorexia. Radiation enteritis may develop into ulceration or obstruction. Radiation depresses the immune system of the body.

Surgery: Resection of the duodenum affects pancreatic and biliary secretion, with malabsorption of various nutrients. Resection of the ileum may cause vitamin B_{12} and bile salt malabsorption. Colonic surgery promotes water and electrolyte loss.

Nutritional Care of the Patient with Cancer:

Eating is encouraged by modifying the food and its presentation. Patients with altered taste acuity may be benefited from the increase in sugar flavorings and seasonings in food preparation. Altered source of protein is needed for patients with meat aversion.

For patients with nausea and vomiting, with abdominal fullness, it is better to take carbohydrates such as bread, cookie, steamed bread. Coke and beer seem to alleviate the symptoms. Lemon and dill pickles appear to curb nausea. The patient should eat slowly, and rest after meal.

For patients with dysphagia and mouth dryness, liquid or moist food facilitates the swallowing process. Acidic lemonade and tomato juice may lead to discomfort of the stomach. Honey may be better.

For patients with diarrhea and intestinal cramps, warm

food can reduce the number of times of diarrhea. Potato, banana and mushroom and food with high potassium content is suitable for patients with diarrhea. Hot food can increase peristalsis, leading to decrease absorption of nutrients. Avoid soft drinks, mineral water, beer or food high in water content. For patients treated with radiation therapy to the small intestine, food and vegetables of high fiber content need to be reduced.

For patients with constipation, it is better to drink lots of water, milk or honey. Fruits and vegetables of high fiber content affect the intestinal micro flora, bile salt metabolism, transit time and fecal bulk.

In general, high protein diet is necessary for patients with colon cancer for repair of the normal tissues. Cell-mediated immunity is depressed when protein and energy intake are severely inadequate.

Vitamin A, B, C, E and inorganic salts can prevent cancer proliferation. Food containing retinoids have protective effect in preventing chemical carcinogenesis in epithelial tissues. Large does of vitamin C may retard collagen breakdown and metastases.

CHINESE HERBS FOR COLON CANCER

In treating colon cancer patients with the Chinese herbs, one must understand the patients well. The Chinese Medical theory consider the constitution of each patient individually even if they have the same diagnosis and symptoms. One must consider the Chinese Differential diagnosis using the tongue and pulse method besides the radiological method of diagnosis.

The Chinese consider the tumor cells can be treated by herbs of the following groups:

1. Eliminating toxin and abscess: This group of herbs can directly or indirectly kill or inhibit the growth of the cancer cells. These herbs have anti-bacterial and antifebrile nature, and can eliminate toxin and abscesses. Some herbs can increase the immunity of the patient by increasing the function of the white blood cells, lymphocytes and macrophages. Some herbs can increase the function of the adrenal cortex, and ACH (Adreno-cortical hormone) can enhance the therapeutical effect of the chemical or radiological radiation.

2. Increasing blood circulation and resolving blood stasis: Blood stasis can be caused by either heat or cold, and by poor blood circulation. So this type of patients will have fixed and chronic pain. This tongue is dark red with purplish spots. This group of herb is usually combined with herbs that can invigorate the circulation of *Qi* (the

vital energy) and with the warming or cooling herbs depending on the constitution of the patient. These herbs can increase metabolism and blood circulation, blood permeability, soften the connective tissues, reduce inflammation and pain. They can also correct the ischemic condition of the tumor cells, and increase the sensitivity to the radiation therapy. Some herbs can increase the proteolytic action of the fibrin, and decrease the stability of the fibrin surrounding the tumor cells. This way, the herbs can destroy the agglutination of the fibrin, increase the blood volume and micro-circulation to the tumor cells. Thus the anti-cancer drugs or herbs, together with the lymphocytes fight against the tumor cells, and increase the immunity of the body.

3. Eliminating phlegm and nodules: These herbs can inhibit the growth of the tumor cells, disperse the mass or nodules of the benign tumors, and decrease the secretion around the malignant tumor cells. These herbs are usually combined with the carminatives or digestives to reduce phlegm.

4. Eliminating tumor and masses: These herbs can kill or inhibit the growth of the tumor cells. Some herbs have purgative action, some are toxic. They are usually combined with herbs that can invigorate the blood circulation. The dosage of the herbs must be controlled during the therapy.

5. Tonification: Because the tumor cells proliferative very rapidly, the body is progressively losing weight. Symptoms of deficiency of *Qi* (vital energy), blood, *Yin* (vital essence) and *Yang* (vital function) are found in the

patients. Deficiency of *Qi* and *Yang* usually indicate the deterioration of the organic functions of the body. Deficiency of *Yin* (vital essence) and blood usually indicate the depletion of blood and fluids in the body. These herbs can increase the immunity of the body and phagocytosis of the tumor cells. Some herbs can enhance the function of the pituitary-adrenal glands. Some can increase the number of cAMP , or regulate the ratio of cAMP and cGMP, and inhibit the growth of the tumor cells.

✵ Da Huang 大黃 (Rhubarb)) (*Radix et Rhizoma Rhei*)

(Fig. 1)

The chemical components of rhubarb are anthraquinone (chrysophanol, emodin, rhein, physcion, aloe-emodin, sennoside A, B, C, D), tannin and mucilage.

Rhubarb is a strong purgative. The effective ingredient is Sennoside A, which is decomposed into sennidine by bacteria in the large intestine. The action of evacuation is increased, leading to defecation. The purgative effect is observed 6-8 hrs after oral intake.

Rhein and emodin can inhibit the growth of ascitic carcinoma, melanoma, lymphosarcoma, breast carcinoma and colon carcinoma. They can inhibit the synthesis of DNA, and the multiplication of cancer cells.

Rhubarb is also used for colon obstruction, constipation, hepatitis, gallstone, hypertension, hypercholesteremia.

3-15 gm. of rhubarb is generally used. For purgative action, the herb is boiled for 15 minutes only. If the process of boiling is over 20 minutes, rhein will be decomposed into free ions, and loose the purgative nature. For anti-tumor action, the herb can be boiled together with the other herbs.

✣ Yi Yi Ren 薏苡仁 (Coix seed, barley, Job's-tear seed) (*Semen Coicis*)

(Fig. 2)

Coix contains coixol, coixenolide, vit. B_1, amino acids, starch, protein, and fatty oil.

Coix has the property of anti-tumor and analgesic. It is anti-pyretic, anti-diuretic, and sedative by counteracting the action of caffeine in the central nervous system.

Coix is effective for carcinoma of the colon, stomach, lung and cervix, chorio-epithelioma, malignant reticulosis. It can increase the cellular and humoral immunity of the body. In animal studies, it has been found to increase (6 times) the hemolytic plague in the spleen. It enhances the function of the adrenal cortex and can diminish the size of the thymus. Some ingredient can stop the mitosis process in the middle phase, and some can change the plasma content of the cancer cells.

Coix is also used for edema, beri-beri, oliguria, diarrhea, rheumatic arthritis, lung and intestinal abscesses.

15-60 gm. of dosage can be used for cancer condition. For normal food preparation, soak 10-30 gm. of the seed overnight to reduce the cooking time.

✘ Bai Hua She She Cao 白花蛇舌草 (Oldenlandia)) (*Herba Oldenlandiae*)

(Fig. 3)

Oldenlandia contains stigmasterol, oleanolic acid, β-sitosterol, *d*-glyside, fatty acid, palmitic acid, oleic acid, linoleic acid, etc.

Oldenlandia is effective for cancer of the colon and digestive tract, liver, cervix, larynx, lymphosarcoma, leukemia (acute granulocytic leukemia, acute lymphocytic leukemia).

The components of oldenlandia can inhibit the mitosis process of the tumor cells, and can cause degeneration and necrosis of the tumor tissues. It can also increase the immunity of the body. There are increases in the function of the reticulo-endothelium system, hypertrophy of the reticulum cells, enrichment of the plasma, increase in the production of white blood cells and antibodies and increase in phagocytosis. There is changes in density of the argentaffin in liver, spleen and lymph nodes. This argentaffin can enwrap the cancer nests, making the infiltration and metastasis more difficulty or impossible.

Oldenlandia is also anti-bacterial, anti-inflammatory, analgesic, and sedative. It can be used for jaundice, tonsillitis, appendicitis, cholecystitis, urinary tract infection, and inflammation of the soft tissues.

The dosage is 30-100 gm. daily. It can be taken orally

or injected, or prepared into tablets, granules, or extracts.

✹ Ku Shen 苦參 (Sophora root, Bitter ginseng) (*Radix Sophorae Flavescentis*)

(Fig. 4)

The chemical components are alkaloids (*d*-matrine, *d*-oxymatrine, *d*-sophoranol, 5-hydroxymatrine, *l*-anagyrine, *l*-methy*l*-cystisine, *l*-baptifoline, *l*-sophocarpine), flavonoid (isoanhydro-icaritin, non-anhydro-icaritin, xanthohumol, isoxanthohumol).

Sophora can be used for cancer of the colon, cervix, skin, soft tissues. Matrine and oxymatrine can increase the production of white blood cells, and the function of reticulo-endothelium system. Sophora is diuretic, antibacterial, anti-fungal, anti-parasitic, and anti-pruritic. It is also used for acute dysentery, leukorrhea, vaginitis, eczema, acute urinary tract infection.

The dosage is 3-10 gm. daily. It can be taken orally, or prepared with other herbs as enema for colon or vagina.

✹ Gua Lou 瓜蔞 (Trichosanthes peel and seed) (*Pericarpium et Semen Trichosanthis*)

(Fig. 5)

The fruit contains triterpene, organic acid, resin, sugar. The seed contains fatty oil, resin and trichosanic acid.

Trichosanthes is used for cancer of the colon, stomach,

lung, pancreas, breast, thyroid, and fibroadenoma. Experiments have confirmed the inhibitory action of trichosanthes against ascites carcinoma and sarcoma. The peel is stronger than the seed in anti-cancer action.

Trichosanthes can dilate the coronary artery and increase the blood flow. It can also increase the tolerance of the body against environmental low blood pressure with decrease oxygen content. Thus it can protect the body against chest pain and acute myocardial ischemic condition. So it is also used for coronary heart disease, pneumonia, bronchitis and abscesses of the colon with constipation.

The dosage is 10-30 gm. daily. It can be taken orally, or prepared into tablets or injections.

⌘ Da Ji 大 薊 (Japanese thistle) (*Herba seu Radix Cirsii Japonici*)

(Fig. 6)

The chemical components of Japanese thistle are taraxasteryl acetate, stigmaterol, α-amyrin, β-amyrin, β-sitosterol.

Cirsium is used for cancer of the lung, colon, liver, cervix, thyroid, urinary bladder and lymphosarcoma. It can increase the hemolytic plaque in the spleen, and the formation of E-rosette. It can increase both the cellular and humoral immunity of the body.

It can also shorten the bleeding time and clotting time, similar to the action of prothrombin. It is also anti-bacterial and anti-hypertensive. So it is used for hypertension, tuberculosis, abscesses, hematuria, and other bleeding or vomiting blood conditions.

The dosage is 15-60 gm. for cancer condition. For ordinary diseases, 10-15 gm. is enough. It can be taken orally or externally.

✘ Ya Dan Zi 鴉膽子 (Brucea fruit) (*Fructus Bruceae*)
(Fig. 7)

The chemical components are alkaloids (brucamarine, yatanine), glucoside (brucealin, yatanoside), phenol (brucenol), bruceolic acid, fatty oil.

Brucea fruit is used for cancer of the lung, skin, colon, rectum, breast, stomach, and esophagus. It can inhibit the growth of spermatocyte. It can cause the karyorrhexis of the nucleus and nuclear membrane, karyopyknosis, vacuolation of the nucleus, and mild nuclear hyperchromatism. Its chloroform extract strongly inhibits the growth of fibrocyte.

Brucea fruit also kills amoebae and plasmodium. It is used for chronic diarrhea, amoebic dysentery, malaria, and trichomonas vaginitis. It is used externally for warts and clavus.

This herb can cause irritation to the G-I tract. It can cause nausea, vomiting, abdominal pain, bloody stool, and may lower the blood pressure.

The recommended dosage is 15-20 pc. (app. 1.5 - 2.0

gm) each time, three times daily. It is crushed into powder form, and put in capsules. It is better to take the herb together with Long Yan Rou (longan). This dosage can be slightly increased for patients with tumor or dysentery. It can also be boiled with water, and used for vaginitis as enema.

✖ Ren Shen 人参 (Ginseng) (*Radix Ginseng*)

(Fig. 8)

The chemical component of ginseng are panaxosides, essential oil (panacene, panaxynol), saponin (ginsenoside), protopanaxadiol, protopanaxatriol. Ginsenoside is Ro, Ra1. Rb is divided into Rb1 and Rb2. These can prevent hemolytic activity caused by natural saponin and lecithin. Rg is divided into Rg1, Rg2, and Rg3.

Ginseng is used for cancer of the colon, cervix, stomach, digestive tract, and leukemia. It increases the immunity of the body. It can increase the production of white blood cells, and immunoglobulin (IgG and IgM). It increases the production of lymphocytes and promote the transformation of lymphoblast.

It increases the synthesis of DNA, RNA, protein and lipid. Ginseng has similar action as the adaptogen, and can increase the defense capabilities of the body. It can regulate the nervous system, cardiovascular system, digestive system, endocrine system, sugar and fat metabolism. It can also reduce fatigue of the body, and improve learning ability of the brain.

Ginseng is usually used in combination with other herbs for cancer or used hand in hand with surgery, chemical therapy and radiation therapy. It can effectively prevent the destruction of white blood cells and other toxic side effects from the radiation and drugs. It can speed up the healing process after surgery, and increase the immunity of the body to kill the remaining tumor cells.

Ginseng is also used for shock and prostration, fatigue, exhaustion, diarrhea, dehydration, insomnia, palpitation, and forgetfulness.

The dosage of ginseng is 3-10 gm. when boiling as decoction. It can be used singly in powder form, 0.3 -0.5 gm. each time, 2-3 times per day. It can also be taken in the tincture form. 5-10 c.c. of the 10% ginseng tincture can be taken each time, 2-3 times daily.

✼ Huang Qi 黃耆 (Astragalus root) (*Radix Astragali*)

Astragalus contains sugars, choline, folic acid, amino acids, β-sitosterol, betaine, astragalan, astragalin.(Fig. 9)

It can be used for tumors of the lung, liver, digestive tract, and all kinds of tumor with asthenia of *Qi* (vital energy) symptoms and weakness.

Astragalus can increase the content of cAMP in the body and inhibit the growth of the tumor cells. It increases the sensitivity to interferon. Interferon is similar to adenylate cyclase in action, can increase the transformation of lymphoblast, increase cAMP, and thus increase immunity. It increases the production of plasma cells and antibody, and has effect against the immunosuppressants. It increases the production of macrophage and thus increase the body resistance. Thus it is effective for both cellular and humoral immunity. It can also increase the number of glycogen granules and mitochondria. It increases the activity of multiple enzymes and the vitality of the body. The polysaccharide have detoxification action on phytohemagglutinin, carbon tetrachloride and prednisolone.

It is also diuretic, cardiotonic, and anti-hypertensive. It prevents the loss of glycogen content in liver. It inhibits the secretion of gastric juice and increases the pH values. Thus it is usually used for edema, diarrhea, prolapse of the uterus, stomach and rectum.

The dosage is 10-30 gm. in decoction.

✘ Bai Zhu 白朮 (White Atractylodes) (Rhizoma Atractylodis Macrocephalae)

It contains atractylone, atractylol, and vit. A.(Fig. 10)

White atractylodes is used for carcinoma of the lung, cervix, digestive tract. It can increase the antigenic and organic specific active immunity of the body. It increases the phagocytosis of bacteria, and enhances the phagocytic capability of the reticulo-endothelium system. It can initiate the formation of E-rosette and the transformation of the lymphoblast. It can also strengthen the function of the pituitary-adrenal cortex.

It is a diuretic, increases the excretion of electrolytes, especially the sodium ions. It can increase the body weight and muscle tone of the body. It enhances the assimilation of glucose and lowers blood sugar. It has anti-coagulant action by increasing the prothrombin time and clotting time. It is used for patients that have edema, dyspepsia, abdominal distention, chronic diarrhea and spontaneous perspiration. The dosage used is 3-15 gm. in decoction.

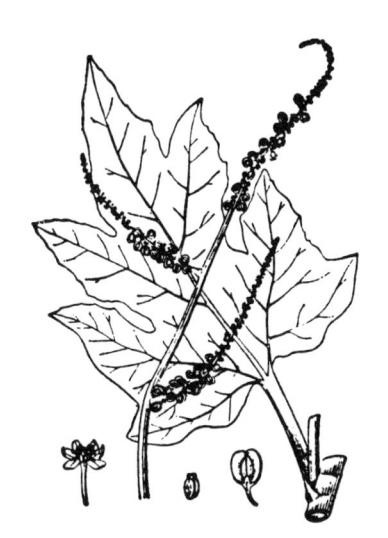

(Fig. 1)

Da Huang 大黄
(Rhubarb)
Radix et Rhizoma Rhei

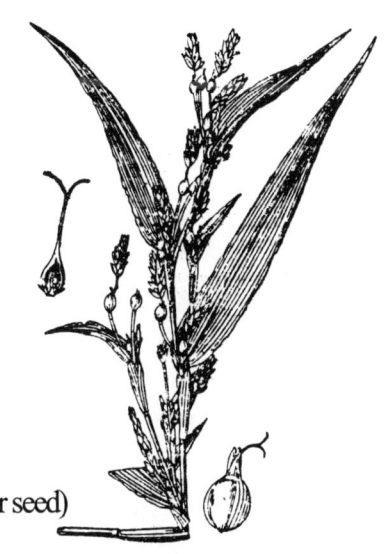

(Fig. 2)

Yi Yi Ren 薏苡仁
(Coix seed, Barley, Job's tear seed)
Semen Coicis

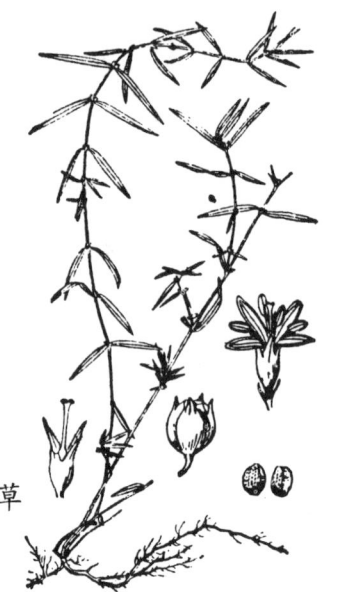

(Fig. 3)

Bai Hua She She Cao 白花蛇舌草
(Oldenlandia)
Herba Oldenlandiae

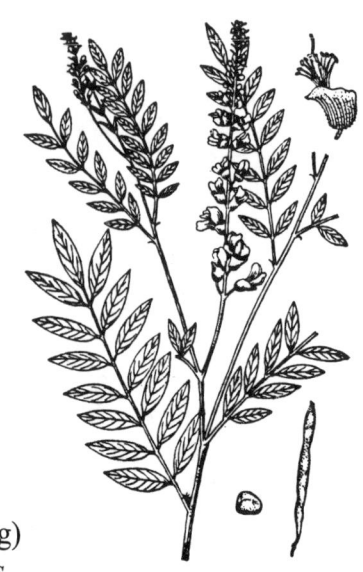

(Fig. 4)

Ku Shen 苦参
(Sophora root, Bitter Ginseng)
Radix Sophorae Flavescentis

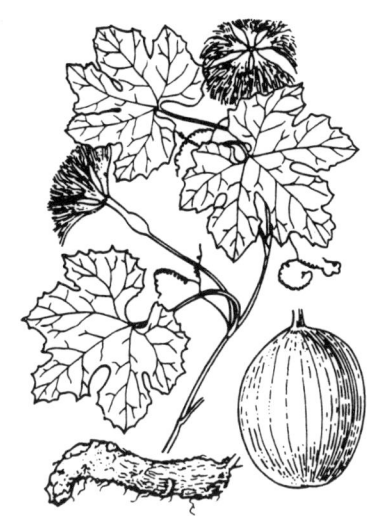

(Fig. 5)

Gua Lou 瓜蔞
(Trichosanthes peel and seed)
Pericarpium et Semen Trichosanthis

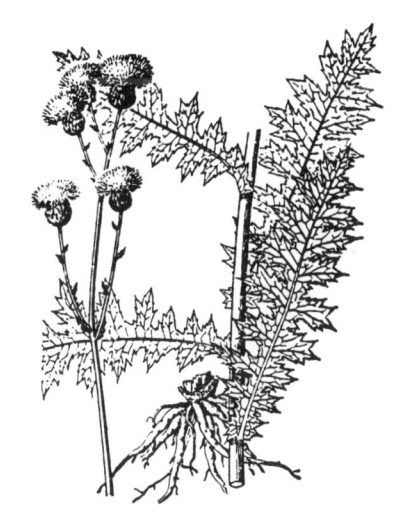

(Fig. 6)

Da Ji 大薊
(Japanese thistle)
Herba seu Radix Cirsii Japonici

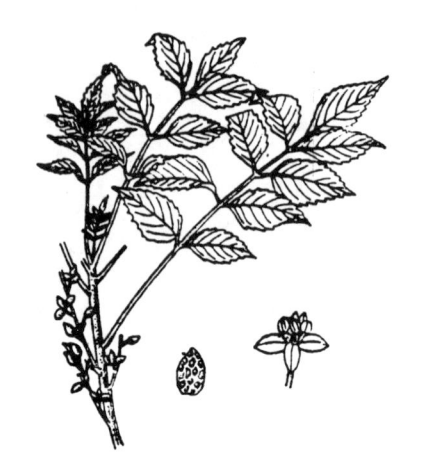

(Fig. 7)
Ya Dan Zi 鴉膽子
(Brucea fruit)
Fructus Bruceae

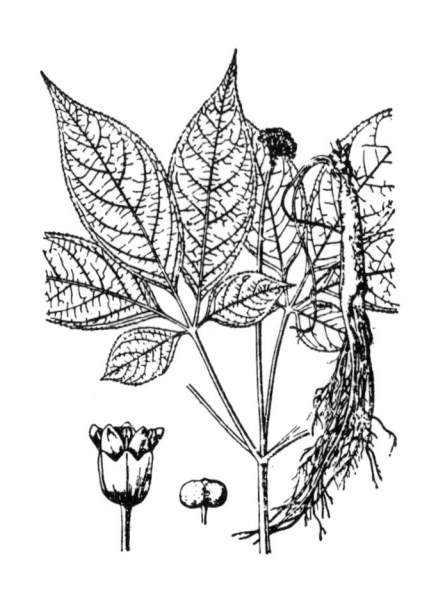

(Fig. 8)
Ren Shen 人參
(Ginseng)
Radix Ginseng

(Fig. 9)

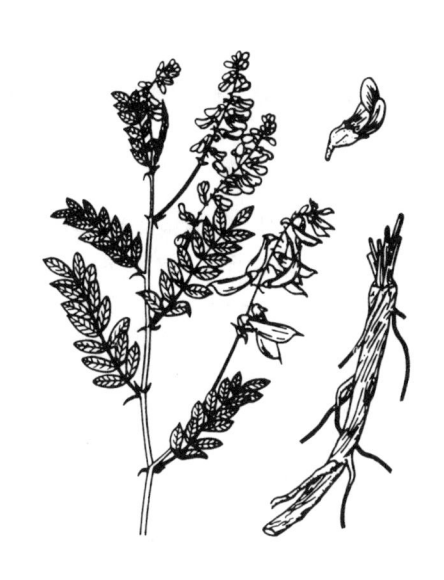

Huang Qi 黄耆
(Astragalus root)
Radix Astragali

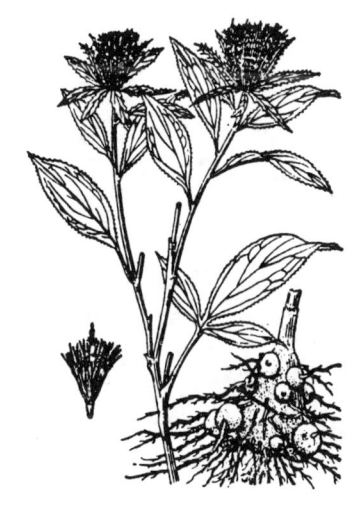

(Fig. 10)

Bai Zhu 白术
(White Astractylodes)
Rhizoma Atractylodis Macrocephalae

Chinese Herbs for Colitis

✻ Shan Yao 山藥 (Chinese yam; Dioscorea) *Rhizoma Dioscoreae)*

(Fig. 11)

The chemical components are starch, mannan, allantoin, arginine, choline, diastase, saponin, mucilage, phytic acid, vitamin C.

Dioscorea is easily digested in the G-I tract, so it can strengthen the function of the spleen and stomach. It is used for chronic diarrhea, leukorrhea, colitis, diabetes, asthma, nocturnal emission and enuresis.

The dosage is 9-30 gm. Fresh and dried dioscorea are commonly used in soup-cooking.

✻ Lian Zi 蓮子 (Lotus seed) (*Semen Nelumbinis)*
(Fig. 12)

Lotus seed contains raffinose, protein, carbohydrates, calcium, phosphorus and iron.

It is a tonic and sedative. It is used in colitis, chronic diarrhea, leukorrhea, insomnia, palpitation, and spontaneous seminal emission.

The dosage is 9-18 gm. Fresh and dried lotus seed are

commonly used in cooking as soup and dessert. It is also available in cans and dry powdered form. Dehydrating the powder makes delicous drinks.

✘ Bai Bian Dou 白扁豆 (Dolichos seed; Hyacinth bean; Egyptian kidney bean) *(Semen Dolichoris Album)*

(Fig. 13)

The chemical components are: hemagglutinin A and B, phytin, protein, fat, carbohydrates, iron, zinc, calcium and phosphorus.

Dolichos bean is used for colitis, vomiting and diarrhea (especially in summer), leukorrhea, and infantile malnutrition. It is capable of prolonging the coagulation time, lowering blood sugar and serum cholesterol.

The usual dosage is 9-18 gm. It is used raw to eliminate summer heat and dampness. It is stir-baked to strengthen the spleen and stomach.

✘ Yi Yi Ren 薏苡仁 (Coix seed, Job's-tears seed) *(Semen Coicis)*

(Fig. 2)

The chemical components are coixol, coixenolide, vitamin B_1, amino acids, starch, protein, and fatty oil.

It is used for colitis with diarrhea, edema, abscessed,

rheumatic arthritis. It is an analgesic, anti-tumor, anti-pyretic and anti-diuretic. It is an excellent grain to take for a long time for beauty and prevent colitis.

The usual dosage is 9-30 gm. It is commonly used for soup preparation and decoction.

✄ Bai Ji 白芨(Bletilla tuber) (*Rhizoma Bletillae*)

(Fig. 14) and front cover

The chemical components are starch, glucose, essential oil, mucilage, (Bletilla glucomnnan).

Bletilla tuber is hemostatic, and anti-inflammatory. It is used for colitis with bleeding, gastric and duodenal ulcer. It is also used for wounds, carbuncles, tuberculosis and suppurative infections.

The hemostatic action is related to the mucilage content. It causes the aggregation of red blood cells on the peripheral blood vessels and the formation of artificial thrombus. It can shorten the coagulation time and prothrombin time. The mucilage can also increase the healing of wounds by granulation.

The usual dosage is 5-15 gm. It can be used internally as decoction, or externally in the powder form.

⌘ Mu Xiang 木 香 (Saussurea root) (*Radix Saussureae)*

(Fig. 15)

The chemical components are essential oil, stigmasterol, betulin, saussurine.

Saussurea is anti-spasmodic, anti-hypertensive and anti-bacterial. It can relieve the abdominal spasm and distention with tenesmus and colitis.

The usual dosage is 3-9 gm. If it is roasted in hot ashes, it can be used for diarrhea.

⌘ Long Yan Rou 龍 眼 肉 (Longan aril) (*Arillus Longan)*

(Fig. 16)

Longan contains glucose, sucrose, protein, choline, adenin and tartaric acid.

It is sweet and nourishing to the body. It is used for chronic colitis with weakness and dehydration.

The usual dosage is 6-12 gm. It can be eaten fresh as fruit or dried.

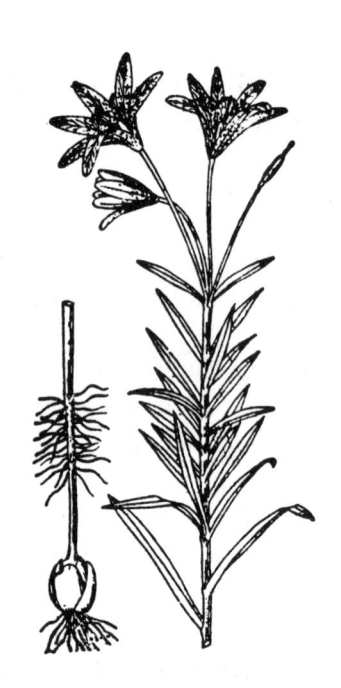

(Fig. 11)

Shan Yao 山藥
(Chinese yam, Dioscorea)
Rhizoma Dioscoreae

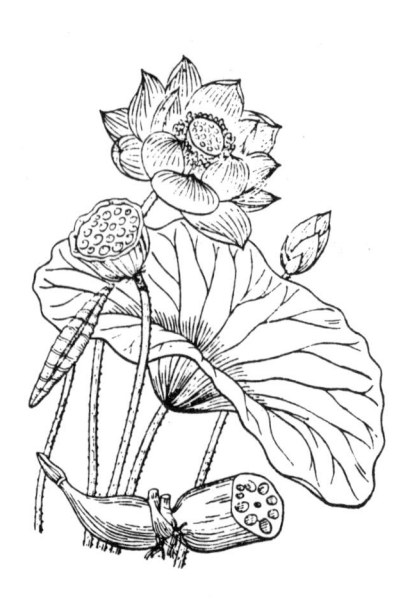

(Fig. 12)

Lian Zi 蓮子
(Lotus seed)
Semen Nelumbinis

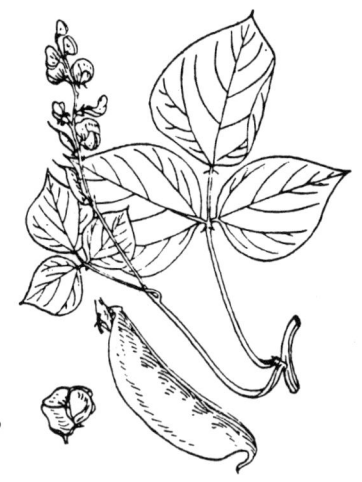

(Fig. 13)

Bai Bian Dou 白扁豆
(Dolichos seed;Hyacinth bean,
Egyptian kidney bean)
Semen Dolichoris Album

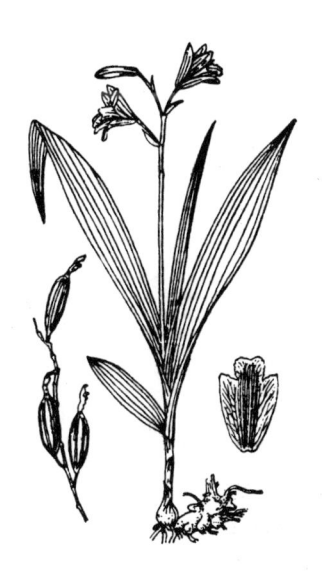

(Fig. 14)

Bai Ji 白芨
(Bletilla tuber)
Rhizoma Bletillae

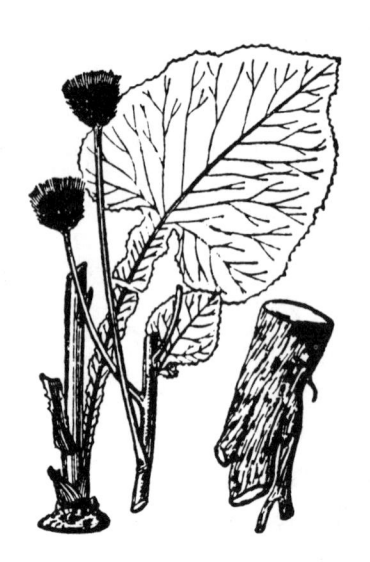

(Fig. 15)

Mu Xiang 木香
(Saussurea root)
Radix Saussureae

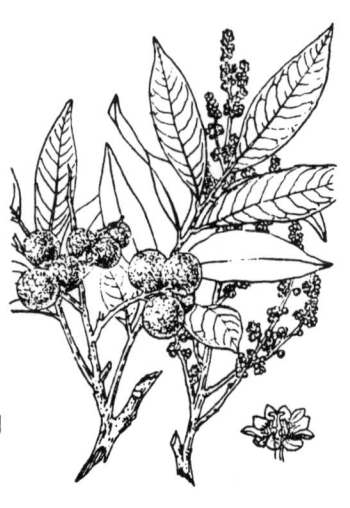

(Fig. 16)

Long Yan Rou 龍眼肉
(Longan aril)
Arillus Longan

Acupuncture Points Used

Zhangmen 章門 (Liv. 13)

Location: On the lateral side of the abdomen, below the free end of the 11th floating rib. (Fig. 17)

Method: Puncture obliquely or perpendicularly 0.8 -1.0 inch. Moxibustion is applicable.

Anatomy: On the right side is the lower margin of the liver and the ascending colon, and on the left side is the descending colon. The muscles involved are the M. obliquus internus abdominis, M. obliquus externus abdominis and M. transversus abdominis. There are lateral cutaneous branches of the 10th and 11th intercostal nerves in the superficial layer. In the deeper layer, there are the 10th and 11th intercostal vessels.

Indications: Vomiting, diarrhea, colitis, indigestion, borborygmus, abdominal distention, jaundice, pain in the chest, lumbar, costal and hypochondriac regions.

Zhongwan 中腕 (Ren 12)

Location: 4 inch above the umbilicus, on the midline of the abdomen. (Fig. 18)

Method: Puncture perpendicularly 1-2 inch. Moxibustion is applicable.

Anatomy: It is located on the linea alba. There are

tributaries of the superior epigastric artery and vein. It is innervated by the anterior cutaneous branches of the 7th and 8th thoracic nerves in the superficial and deep layer.

Indications: Gastric pain, abdominal distention, regurgitation, vomiting, diarrhea, colitis, dysentery, gastritis, gastric ulcer, gastric ptosis, dyspepsia, acute intestinal obstruction.

Tianshu 天樞 (St. 25)

Location: 2 inch lateral to the umbilicus. (Fig. 18)

Method: Puncture perpendicularly 1-2 inch. Moxibustion is applicable.

Anatomy: It is located on the M. rectus abdominis and its sheath. There are the superficial and inferior epigastric arteries and veins. It is innervated by the cutaneous branches of the 10th intercostal nerve in the superficial layer.

Indications: Abdominal pain, colitis, diarrhea, constipation, borborygmus, abdominal distention, dysentery, gastritis, enteritis, and appendicitis.

Shenjue 神闕 (Ren 8)

Location: In the center of the umbilicus. (Fig. 18)

Method: This point should not be punctured. Moxibustion is done with a moxa-stick for 5-15 minutes, or with a moxa-cone (5-15 in number) on top of a thin layer of salt or a slice of ginger or aconite.

Anatomy: The deep part of this point are omentum majus and intestinum tenue. There are the anterior cutaneous branches of the 10th thoracic nerve, and the inferior epigastric artery and vein.

Indications: Acute and chronic enteritis, colitis, chronic dysentery, borborygmus, diarrhea, abdominal distention, edema, intestinal tuberculosis, flaccid type of apoplexy.

Qihai 氣海 (Ren 6)

Location: 1.5 inch below the umbilicus, on the midline of the abdomen. (Fig. 18)

Method: Puncture perpendicularly 0.8-1.2 inch. Moxibustion may be applied often.

Anatomy: In the deep part are the omentum majus and intestinum tenue. There are superficial epigastric artery and vein. It is innervated by the anterior cutaneous branches of the 11th and 12th thoracic nerves in the superficial and deep layer.

Indications: Irregular menstruation, dysmenorrhea, postpartum hemorrhage, abdominal pain, irregular uterine bleeding, prolapse of the uterus, hernia, enuresis, constipation, impotence, diarrhea, colitis, frequent micturition, retention of urine, edema, flaccid type of apoplexy.

Comment: This is one of the important points for tonification.

Guanyuan 關元 (Ren 4)

Location: 3 inch below the umbilicus, on the midline of the umbilicus. (Fig. 18)

Method: Puncture needle perpendicularly 1-1.5 inch. Moxibustion may be applied fairly long and frequently.

Anatomy: In the deep part are the intestinum tenue and omentum majus. In the superficial layer are the branches of the superficial epigastric vessels. In the deep layer are the branches of the inferior epigastric vessels. It is innervated by the medial branches of the anterior cutaneous subcostal nerve.

Indications: Irregular menstruation, dysmenorrhea, amenorrhea, leukorrhea, infertility, uterine bleeding, prolapse of the uterus, postpartum hemorrhage, hernia, lower abdominal pain, diarrhea, colitis, impotence, early ejaculation, spermatorrhea, enuresis, retention of urine, frequent urination, dripping of urine, etc.

Dazhui 大椎 (Du 14)

Location: Between the spinous processes of the 7th cervical vertebra and the first thoracic vertebra. (Fig. 19)

Method: Puncture perpendicularly or obliquely 0.5-1 inch slightly upward.

Anatomy: It is located at the fascia lumbodorsalis supraspinal and interspinal ligaments. There are branches of the transverse cervical artery, and the interspinal venous plexus. It is innervated by the posterior ramus of the 8th cervical nerve, and the medial branch of the posterior ramus of the first thoracic nerve.

Indication: Fever, malaria, common cold, cough, asthma, urticaria, stiff neck and back, weakness.

Comment: This is a tonic point. Used for prevention of diseases and promotion of health.

Pishu 脾俞 (U.B. 20)

Location: 1.5 inch lateral to the lower border of the spinous process of the 11th thoracic vertebra. (Fig. 19)

Method: Puncture perpendicularly 0.5-1 inch or obliquely toward the vertebra columm. Moxibustion is applicable.

Anatomy: It is located on M. latissimus dorsi, M. longissimus and M. iliocostalis. It is supplied by the branches of the 11th intercostal artery and vein. In the superficial layer, there are the medial cutaneous branches of the posterior rami of the 11th and 12th thoracic nerves. In the deeper layer, there are the lateral branches.

Indications: Abdominal distention, jaundice, vomiting, colitis, diarrhea, dysentery, edema, indigestion, back pain.

Comment: This is the Back-shu point of the spleen.

Weishu 胃俞 (U.B. 21)

Location: 1.5 inch lateral to the lower border of the spinous process of the 12th thoracic vertebra. (Fig. 19)

Method: Puncture perpendicularly 0.5 -1 inch or obliquely toward the vertebral column. Moxibustion is applicable.

Anatomy: It is located on the fascia lumbodorsalis, M. longissimus and M. iliocostalis. It is supplied by the medial branches of the posterior branches of the subcostal artery and vein. In the superficial layer, there are the medial cutaneous branches of the posterior ramus of the 12th thoracic nerve. In the deeper layer, there are the lateral branches.

Locations: Pain in the chest, hypochondriac and epigastric region, abdominal distention, colitis, regurgitation, nausea, vomiting, borborygmus, indigestion, chronic diarrhea.

Comment: This is the Back-shu point of the stomach.

Shenshu 肾俞 (U.B. 23)

Location: 1.5 inch lateral to the lower border of the spinous process of the 2nd lumbar vertebra. (Fig. 19)

Method: Puncture perpendicularly 0.5-1 inch, or obliquely toward the vertebral column. Moxibustion is applicable.

Anatomy: It is located on the fascia lumbodorsalis, M. longissimus and M. iliocostalis. It is supplied by the medial branches of the posterior branches of the 2nd lumbar artery and vein. It is innervated by the lateral cutaneous branch of the posterior ramus of the first lumbar nerve in the superficial layer, and the lateral branches in the deeper layer.

Indications: Low back pain, seminal emission, impotence, enuresis, retention of urine, irregular menstruation, leukorrhea, weakness of the knee, blurring of vision, tinnitus, deafness, edema, chronic diarrhea, colitis, shortness of breath due to weakness of kidney.

Comment: This is the Back-shu point of the kidney.

Dachangshu 大腸俞 (U.B. 25)

Location: 1.5 inch lateral to the lower border of the spinous process of the 4th lumbar vertebra, approximately at the level of the upper border of the iliac crest. (Fig. 19)

Method: Puncture perpendicularly 1-1.5 inch or obliquely toward the vertebral column. Moxibustion is applicable.

Anatomy: It is located on the fascia lumbodorsalis superficially, and on the M. sacrospinalis in the deeper layer. It is supplied by the medial branch of the posterior branch of the 4th lumbar artery and vein. It is innervated by the posterior ramus of the 3rd lumbar nerve.

Indications: Acute and chronic low back pain, sciatica, neuralgia, colitis, constipation, diarrhea, borborygmus, abdominal pain and distention.

Comment: This is the Back-shu point of the large intestine.

Mingmen 命門 (Du 4)

Location: Between the spinous process of the 2nd and 3rd vertebrae. (Fig. 19)

Method: Puncture needle perpendicularly 0.5-1.5 inch.

Moxibustion is applicable.

Anatomy: It is located on the fascia lumbodorsalis, supraspinal and interspinal ligaments. It is supplied by the posterior branch of the lumbar artery, and the subcutaneous interspinal venous plexus. It is innervated by the medial branch of the posterior ramus of the lumbar nerve.

Indications: Impotence, seminal emission, menorrhalgia, irregular menstruation, leukorrhea, colitis, chronic diarrhea, low back pain.

Caution: Care must be taken in puncturing the points above the spinous process of the second lumbar vertebra. Don't puncture too deep so as to avoid injuring the spinal medulla.

Zusanli 足 三 里 (St.. 36)

Location: 3 inch below the patella, lateral to the patella ligament, one finger width lateral to the anterior crest of the tibia. (Fig. 20)

Method: Puncture perpendicularly 1-2 inch, or obliquely downward 2-3 inch. Moxibustion is applicable.

Anatomy: It is located between the tibia and fibula. It is located on the M. anterior tibialis and M. extensor digitorum longus. It is supplied by the anterior tibial artery and vein. There are branches of the lateral sural nerve and the cutaneous branch of the saphenous nerve in the superficial layer; and the deep peroneal nerve in the deep layer.

Indications: Gastritis, peptic ulcer, pancreatitis, diarrhea, enteritis, colitis, stomachache, borborygmus, constipation, bacillary dysentery, abdominal distention, nausea and vomiting, diseases of the digestive tract, diseases of the knee joint and the anterior aspect of the lower extremity.

Comment: This point is also called the longevity point of the body. It is used for promotion of health and prevention of diseases.

Shangjuxu 上巨虛 (St.. 37)

Location: 3 inch below Zusanli, or 6 inch below the lateral side of the patella, one finger breadth from the anterior crest of the tibia. (Fig. 20)

Method: Puncture needle perpendicularly 0.5-1.5 inch. Moxibustion is applicable.

Anatomy: It is located in the space between the tibia and fibula. It is located on the M. tibialis anterior. It is supplied by the anterior tibial artery and vein. There are branches of the lateral sural cutaneous nerve, and the cutaneous branch of the saphenous nerve in the superficial layer. In the deeper layer is the deep peroneal nerve.

Indications: Abdominal pain and distention, borborygmus, diarrhea, colitis, dysentery, appendicitis, beriberi, hemiplegia, diseases of the lower extremities.

Hegu 合谷 (L.I. 4)

Location: Between the 1st and 2nd metacarpal bones, at the highest point of the 1st M. interosseous dorsalis. (Fig. 21)

Method: Puncture perpendicularly 0.5-1 inch.

Anatomy: Underneath is the 1st M. interosseous dorsalis and M. adductor pollicis. It is supplied by the venous network of the dorsum of the hand. In the superficial layer there are the dorsal vein of the hand, and the superficial branches of the radial nerve. In the deeper layer is the digital palmar proprial nerve from the median nerve.

Indications: Abdominal pain, toothache, tonsillitis, common cold, facial paralysis, hemiplegia.

Comment: This point is most effective for the relief of pain. It is used to obtain acupuncture anesthesia for many purposes.

Zhangmen (Liv. 13)

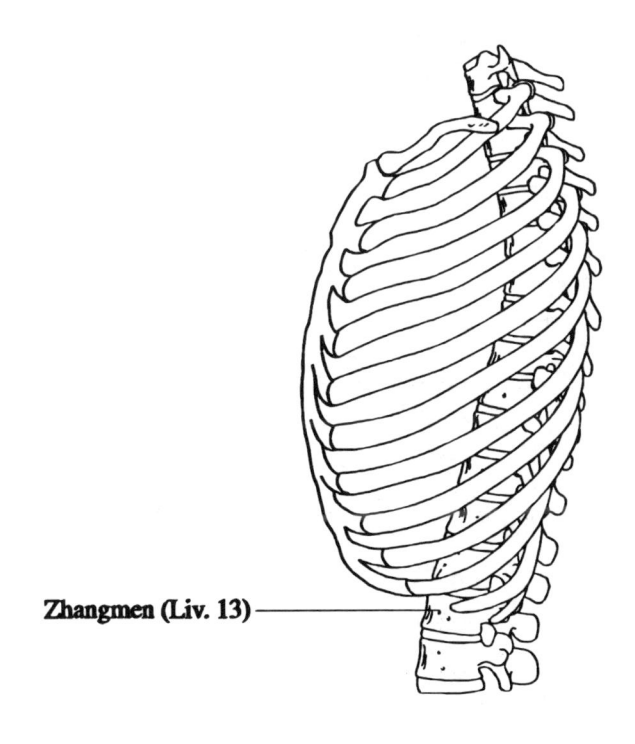

Figure 17

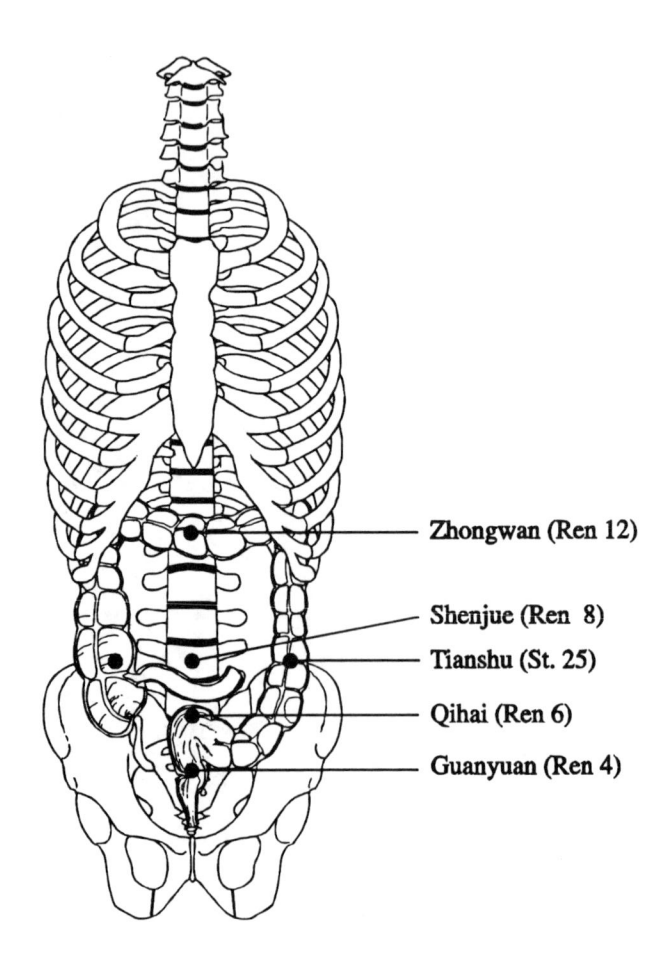

Figure 18

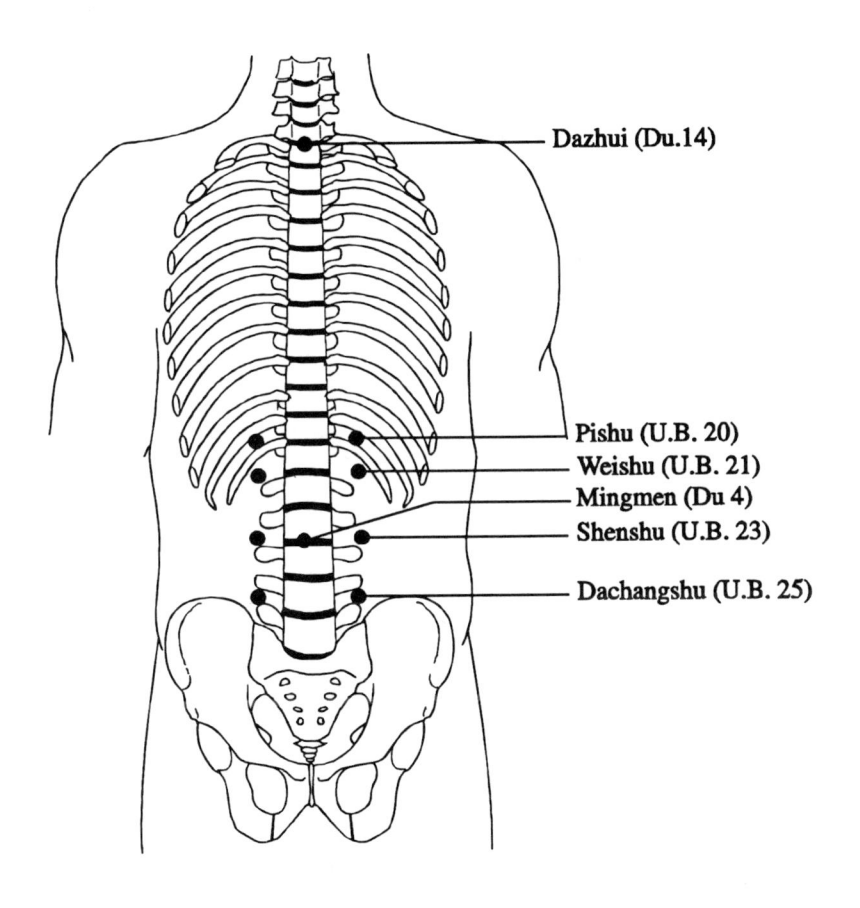

Figure 19

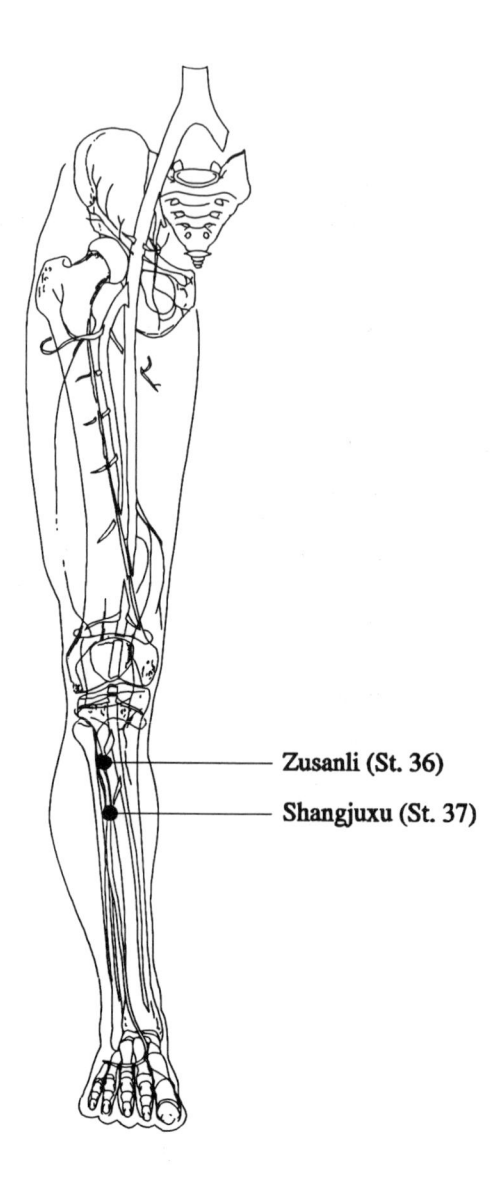

Figure 20

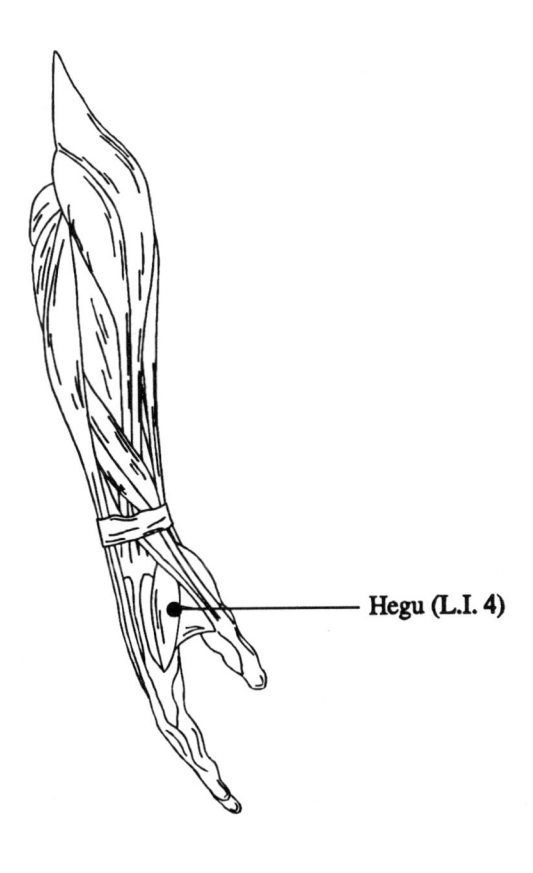

Figure 21

GLOSSARY

Decoction 湯藥

The herb broth obtained by boiling the ingredients of the herbal formulas with appropriate amount of water in a clay pot for a period of time. The herbs are decanted, and the broth is taken usually after meal.

Deficiency of Yin 陰虛

A morbid state of the body due to the deficiency of *Yin* - fluid. The symptoms are low-graded or afternoon fever, face flushed red, lips red, dry mouth, night sweat, warmth in the palms and soles, scanty and dark urine. Tongue red with thin coating, and pulse thready and rapid.

Deficiency of Yang 陽虛

A morbid state of the body due to the insufficiency of *Yang* . The symptoms are fatigue, lack of energy, face pale, cold hands and feet, spontaneous perspiration, loose stools, increase in urine excretion. Tongue pale, and pulse weak.

Insufficiency of spleen and kidney Yang 脾腎陽虛

A morbid state of the body due to the insufficiency of spleen *Yang* which controls the transportation and transformation of the food products and the heat energy required to carry on the process. The loss of heat energy will lead to diarrhea and cold limbs. The insufficiency of kidney *Yang* will also lead to cold limbs, aversion to cold, low back pain, impotence, nocturia, spermatorrhea and weakness in both knees.

Liver Qi 肝氣

The vital energy and functional activities of the liver. An upset of the liver *Qi* will lead to dyspepsia, irritability, distension and pain in the hypochrondric region, oppression in the chest, and irregular menstruation.

Ming-men 命門

The fire from the Gate of Life. It is located between the two kidneys, between the first and second spinous process of the lumbar vertebra. The function is the same as the kidney *Yang*. This acupuncture point is used for treatment of impotence, low back pain, spermatorrhea, leukorrhea, and chronic diarrhea.

Qi 氣

The vital energy or functional activity of the energy. It includes the respiratory circulation of oxygen and carbon dioxide, and the flow of nutritive substances such as water, electrolytes, glucose and other end products of food (fat, protein and carbohydrates). The flow of *Qi* is from organ to organ, and also follows the pattern of flow of the meridians of the body.

Yin-Yang 陰陽

A general term for two opposite aspects of matters in nature. Yet they are interrelated with each other. Generally, *Yin* is the vital essence, and *Yang* is the vital function.

Generally, inhalation is *Yang*, and exhalation is *Yin*.

The Sympathetic nervous system is *Yang*, and the Parasympathetic nervous system is *Yin*.

Metallic ions such as Na, K, Ca, Mg are considered as *Yang*, and non-metallic ions such as Cl, S, P are *Yin*. Alkaline is *Yang*, and acid is *Yin*.

In relation to the body: upper, left, dorsal, exterior are *Yang*, lower, right, ventral, interior are *Yin*. The extensor muscles are *Yang*, the flexor muscles are *Yin*.

In relation to the blood: increase of fat, glucose, ATP, BUN, red blood cell, neutrophils, monocytes, and decrease of platelet are *Yang*; increase of eosinophils, basophils, T- and B-lymphocytes are *Yin*.

An imbalance of *Yin* and *Yang* will lead to inequilibrium, leading to relative excessiveness or deficiency, which may then cause disorders of *Qi* and blood.

DISEASES OF THE COLON AND RECTUM

Self-assessment Workbook

1. The stools are frequent, formed, small, but associated with increased urge to defecate.

A. Diarrhea

B. Malabsorption

C. Tenesmus

D. Ulceration

2. The stools are large, oily, malodorous, soft-formed, but no urgency.

A. Diarrhea

B. Malabsorption

C. Tenesmus

D. Ulceration

3. The stools are frequent, voluminous, and poorly formed, no urgency.

A. Diarrhea

B. Malabsorption

C. Tenesmus

D. Ulceration

4. In Crohn's disease, the prime indication for operation are complications of:

A. Stricture

B. Abscess

C. Fistula

D. All of the above

E. None of the above

5. Both colitic arthritis and rheumatoid arthritis do not have which one of the following:

A. Swelling, redness, and limitation of motion of the joints

B. Involvement of the ankles and knees.

C. Have joint deformity

D. Positive rheumatoid factor

E. Birefringent crystals in the joint fluid

6. Chronic ulcerative colitis has the following manifestations, except:

A. Pseudopolyps

B. Fistula

C. Bleeding

D. Micro abscess

7. Granulomatous colitis has the following manifestations, except:

A. Pseudopolyps

B. Fistula

C. Abscess

D. Fissures

8. Diverticulitis of the colon has the following manifestations, except:

A. Perforation

B. Abscess

C. Fistula

D. Common in the sigmoid colon

9. In patients with diarrhea, physiologic studies of the colon tend to show

A. Increased number of contractions

B. Decreased number of contractions

10. Constipation is usually found in the cancer of colon.

A. Cancer of the right colon

B. Cancer of the left colon

C. Cancer of the rectum

D. Cancer of the anus

11. Diarrhea can be caused by the infestation of the following bacterial or parasite, except:

A. Shigella

B. Schistosoma

C. Staphylococcus

D. Entamoeba histolytica

12. Patients with ulcerative colitis usually has hypoproteinemia due to:

A. Malabsorption of protein in the intestines

B. Indigestion of protein

C. Decreased synthesis of protein

D. Loss of protein and decrease in absorption of protein in the inflammatory area

13. The organ that is involved in diarrhea according to the Chinese medical theory are:

A. Spleen, kidney and liver

B. Spleen, kidney and lung

C. Spleen, stomach and liver

D. Kidney, stomach and lung

14. The cause of diarrhea according to the Chinese medical theory is:

A. Earth is not warmed by the fire

B. Earth is weak, and is over-countered by the Wood

C. Spleen is weak, and excess of Dampness

D. Spleen is weak, and excess of Blood

15. Which one of the following is not used for a person with diarrhea, abdominal pain, stool brown and with foul odor, burning sensation in the anus, tongue yellow and greasy, pulse rapid.

A. Huang Lian 黃連 (Coptis) *Rhizoma Coptidis*

B. Bai Shao 白芍 (White peony) *Radix Paeoniae Alba*

C. Lian Zi 蓮子 (Lotus seed) *Semen Nelumbinis*

D. Huang Bai 黃柏 (Phellodendron) *Cortex Phellodendri*

16. Which one of the following is not considered as an astringent herb in control of chronic diarrhea:

A. Bing Lan 檳榔 (Areca seed) *Semen Arecae*

B. He Zi 訶子 (Terminalis fruit) *Fructus Terminaliae*

C. Rou Dou Kou 肉豆蔻 (Nutmeg) *Semen Myristicae*

D. Wu Mei 烏梅 (Mume) *Fructus Mume*

17. Which one of the following is not used for a person with chronic diarrhea (especially in the early morning), pain relieved after bowel movement, low back pain, cold extremities, tongue pale with thin white coat, pulse deep and weak.

A. Fu Zi 附子 (Aconite) *Radix Aconiti Praeparata*

B. Gan Jiang 干姜 (Dry ginger) *Rhizoma Zingiberis*

C. Dang Gui 當歸 (Chinese Angelica) *RadixAngelicaeSinensis*

D. Bu Gu Zhi 補骨脂 (Psoralea) *Fructus Psoraleae*

18. Which one of the following herb is a strong purgative. Prolonged boiling or habitual use will lose its purgative action.

A. Dang Gui 當歸(Chinese Angelica) *Radix Angelicae*

B. Da Huang 大黄 (Rhubarb) *Radix et Rz. Rhei*

C. Gua Lou Ren 瓜蔞仁 (Trichosanthes seed) *Semen*

D. Ku Shen 苦參 (Sophora root) *Radix Sophorae*

19. The following herbs have anti-cancer activity, except:

A. Bai Hua She She Cao 白花蛇舌草(Oldenlandia) *Herba Oldenlandiae*

B. Ban Zhi Lian 半枝蓮(Barbat skullcap) *Herba Scutellariae*

C. Bai Jiang Cao 敗醬草 (Patrinia) *Herba Patriniae*

D. Hong Hua 紅花 (Safflower) *Flos Carthami*

20. Which one of the following points is used for abdominal pain of all kinds.

A. Mingmen 命門 (Du 4)

B. Hegu 合谷(L.I. 4)

C. Zusanli 足三里 (St. 36)

D. Shangjuxu 上巨虛 (St. 37)

21. Which one of the following points is used for relief of pain and is used to obtain acupuncture anesthesia:

A. Guanyuan 關元(Ren 4)

B. Hegu 合谷 (L.I. 4)

C. Zusanli 足三里 (St. 36)

D. Shangjuxu 上巨虛 (St. 37)

22. Which one of the following points is located on the lateral side of the abdomen, below the free end of the 11th floating rib:

A. Tianshu 天樞 (St. 25)

B. Shenjue 神闕 (Ren 8)

C. Zhongwan 中腕 (Ren 12)

D. Zhangmen 章門 (Liv. 13)

23. Which one of the following point is not innervated by the thoracic nerve:

A. Dazhui 大椎 (Du 14)

B. Mingmen 命門 (Du 4)

C. Pishu 脾俞 (U.B. 20)

D. Weishu 胃俞 (U.B. 21)

24. Which one of the following herbal formulas is used for a patient with diarrhea with dark purplish blood,

abdominal distention with sharp pain, non-movable mass, tongue purplish with blood spots, and pulse is hesitant.

A. Shen Ling Bai Zhu San 參苓白朮散

B. Zhi Bai Di Huang Wan 知柏地黃丸

C. Huai Jiao Wan 槐角丸

D. Ge Xia Zhu Yu Tang 膈下逐瘀湯

25. Which one of the following herb is not sweet, and is not used for cooking purposes.

A. Lian Zi 蓮子 (Lotus seed) *Semen Nelumbinis*

B. Long Yan Rou 龍眼肉 (Longan) *Arillus Longan*

C. Bai Ji 白芨 (Bletilla tuber) *Rhizoma Bletillae*

D. Da Zao 大棗 (Jujube) *Fructus Ziziphus Jujubae*

26. Large doses of vitamin C is used for cancer patients because:

A. Can retard collagen breakdown and metastases

B. Can decrease diarrhea and intestinal cramps

C. Can increase peristalsis

D. Can increase cell-mediated immunity

27. Which one of the following drug is used for patients with colorectal cancer before operation:

A. Prednisone

B. 5-Fluouracil

C. Penicillin

D. Sulfasalazine

28. Which one of the following is not used to restore the normal flora in the intestines:

A. Milk

B. Yogurt

C. Acidophilus

D. Whey powder

29. Which one of the following is used as bulk additives:

A. Banana

B. Honey

C. Psyllium seed

D. Oatmeal

30. Which one of the following minerals is decreased in soil leading to increased incidence of colon cancer:

A. Potassium

B. Magnesium

C. Phosphorus

D. Selenium

Answers
(Diseases of the Colon and Rectum)

1. C	16. A
2. B	17. C
3. A	18. B
4. D	19. D
5. E	20. C
6. B	21. B
7. A	22. D
8. C	23. B
9. B	24. D
10. B	25. C
11. C	26. A
12. D	27. B
13. A	28. A
14. C	29. C
15. C	30. D

INDEX

5
5-Fluouracil, 33

A
Adaptogen, 47
Adreno-cortical hormone, 39
Anemia
    microcytic, 4
Anticholinergic, 25
Argentaffin, 43
Astragalus root, 48
Atractylodes, white, 49

B
Ba Zhen Tang, 32
Bai Bian Dou, 57, 60
Bai Hua She She Cao, 43, 52
Bai Ji, 58, 61
Bai Tou Weng Tang, 8
Bai Zhu, 49, 55
Barley, 42
Bletilla, 58
Bran, 25
Brucea, 46

C
cAMP, 41
Carbon tetrachloride, 49
Carcinoma
    anus, 28

    medullary, 27
    rectum, 28
Carcinoma of colon
    chemotherapy, 33
    herbs, 39
    nutrition, 36, 37
    radiation therapy, 33
    treatment, 28
    Treatment (Chinese), 29
Carcinoma of the colon, 26
Carcioma of colon
    diagnosis (Chinese), 29
    therapy (integrated), 34
cGMP, 41
Chinese Diet Therapy, 19
Cirsium, 45
Coix, 57
Colitis
    acupuncture, 13
    enema (Chinese), 12
    fulminant, 3
    granulomatous, 5
    herbs, 56
    nutrition, 17
    pathogenesis (Chinese), 6
    prevention, 16
    treatment, 15
    treatment (Chinese), 7
    ulcerative, 2
Crohn's disease, 5

D

Da Huang, 41
Da Ji, 45, 53
Dachangshu (U.B. 25), 35, 69

Dazhui (Du 14), 66
Dioscorea, 56
Diverticulitis, 24
    symptoms, 24
    treatment, 25
Dolichos, 57
Dysentery
    amoebic, 4
    bacillary, 4
    Shigella, 4

E
Emodin, 41

F
Fibrin, 40
Fibrocarcinoma, 27
Fu Zi Li Zhong Wan, 11
Fulguration, 33

G
Ginseng, 47
Gua Lou, 44, 53
Guanyuan (Ren 4), 36, 66

H
Hegu (L.I. 4), 36, 72
Huang Qi, 48, 55
Hypoproteinemia, 4

I
Interferon, 48

J
Japanese thistle, 45

K
Karyopyknosis, 46

Karyorrhexis, 46
Ku Shen, 44, 52

L

Lian Zi, 56, 60
Long Yan Rou, 59, 62
Longan, 59
Lotus seed, 56

M

Metastasis, 28
Ming Fan He Ji, 13
Mingmen (Du 4), 70
Modified Ge Xia Zhu Yu Tang, 31
Modified Huai Jiao Wan, 29
Mu Xiang, 58, 62
Mucilage, 58

O

Oldenlandia, 43

P

Phytohemagglutinin, 49
Pishu (U.B. 20), 36, 67
Prednisone, 23
Prothrombin, 45
Pseudopolyps, 3
pseudopolyps, 4
Psyllium seed, 25

Q

Qihai (Ren 6), 65

R

Recto-fistula, 28
Ren Shen, 47, 54
Resection, 28
Rhein, 41

Rhubarb, 41

S

Saussurea, 58
Schistosomiasis, 5
Shan Yao, 56, 59
Shangjuxu (St. 37), 35, 71
Shao Fu Zhu Yu Tang, 12
Shen Ling Bai Zhu San, 9, 31
Shenjue (Ren 8), 64
Shenshu (U.B. 23), 35, 68
Si Mo Yin, 10
Si Shen Wan, 11, 31
Sophora root, 44
Sulfasalazine, 23

T

Tianshu (St. 25), 64
Tong Xie Yao Fang, 10
Tonification, 40
Total parenteral nutrition, 17
Trichosanthes, 44

W

Weishu (U.B. 21), 68

Y

Ya Dan Zi, 46, 54
Yi Yi Ren, 42, 57, 61
Yun Nan Bai Yao, 13

Z

Zhangmen (Liv. 13), 63
Zhi Bai Di Huang Wan, 31
Zhongwan (Ren 12), 63
Zusanli (St. 36), 70